Empirically Based Assessment of Child and Adolescent Psychopathology

Developmental Clinical Psychology and Psychiatry Series

Series Editor: Alan E. Kazdin, Yale University

Recent volumes in this series . . .

Empirically Based Assessment of Child and Adolescent Psychopathology
Practical Applications

Second Edition

Thomas M. Achenbach
Stephanie H. McConaughy

Volume 13
Developmental Clinical Psychology and Psychiatry

SAGE Publications
International Educational and Professional Publisher
Thousand Oaks   London   New Delhi

For information address:

SAGE Publications, Inc.
2455 Teller Road
Thousand Oaks, California 91320
E-mail: order@sagepub.com

SAGE Publications Ltd.
6 Bonhill Street
London EC2A 4PU
United Kingdom

SAGE Publications India Pvt. Ltd.
M-32 Market
Greater Kailash I
New Delhi 110 048 India

Printed in the United States of America

Library of Congress Cataloging-in-Publication Data

Achenbach, Thomas M., 1940–
    Empirically based assessment of child and adolescent psychopathology: practical applications / Thomas M. Achenbach, Stephanie H. McConaughy. — 2nd ed.
        p.   cm. — (Developmental clinical psychology and psychiatry; vol. 13)
        Includes bibliographical references (pp. 207-216) and indexes.
        ISBN 0-8039-7247-4 (cloth : acid-free paper). — ISBN
    0-8039-7248-2 (pbk. : acid-free paper)
        1. Behavioral assessment of children. 2. Behavioral assessment of teenagers. 3. Child psychopathology—Case studies. 4. Adolescent psychopathology—Case studies.
    I. McConaughy, Stephanie H.   II. Title.   III. Series: Developmental clinical psychology and psychiatry; v. 13.
    RJ503.5.A33 1996
    618.92′89—dc20   96-10137

97 98 99   10 9 8 7 6 5 4 3 2 1

This book is printed on acid-free paper.

Acquiring Editor:	Jim Nageotte
Production Editor:	Diana E. Axelsen
Production Assistant:	Karen Wiley
Typesetter/Designer:	Christina M. Hill
Print Buyer:	Anna Chin

CONTENTS

LIST OF TABLES

LIST OF FIGURES

LIST OF ACRONYMS

ADHD	Attention Deficit Hyperactivity Disorder
BASC	Behavior Assessment System for Children
BIS	Behavioral Inhibition System
CAS	Child Assessment Schedule
CBCL/2-3	Child Behavior Checklist for Ages 2-3
CBCL/4-18	Child Behavior Checklist for Ages 4-18
CD	Conduct Disorder
CDI	Children's Depression Inventory
CMHC	Community Mental Health Center
CPRS	Conners Parent Rating Scale
CSI	Children's Somatization Inventory
CTAB	Comprehensive Test of Adaptive Behavior
CTRS	Conners Teacher Rating Scale
DISC	Diagnostic Interview Schedule for Children
DOF	Direct Observation Form
DSM	*Diagnostic and Statistical Manual of Mental Disorders*
GDS	Gordon Diagnostic System
HMO	Health Maintenance Organization
ICD	*International Classification of Diseases*
IDEA	Individuals with Disabilities Education Act

IEP	Individualized Education Program
MDT	Multidisciplinary Team
ODD	Oppositional Defiant Disorder
REW	Reward System
RCMAS	Revised Children's Manifest Anxiety Scale
ROC	Receiver Operating Characteristic
SCICA	Semistructured Clinical Interview for Children and Adolescents
SED	Serious Emotional Disturbance
SSRS	Social Skills Rating System
TCRF/2-5	Teacher/Caregiver Report Form for Ages 2-5
TRF	Teacher's Report Form
WJPB-R	Woodcock Johnson Psychoeducational Battery-Revised
YSR	Youth Self-Report

PREFACE

In the first edition of this book (Achenbach & McConaughy, 1987), we illustrated practical applications of our approach to assessment of child and adolescent psychopathology. This approach involves obtaining data on specific behavioral and emotional problems from multiple sources, performing statistical analyses to identify syndromes of co-occurring problems, and constructing profiles for displaying results for individual children in relation to percentiles and standard scores derived from relevant reference groups of peers. When appropriate, children's competencies are also scored on scales for comparison with peers.

Since the first edition of this book, our approach to empirically based assessment has advanced in many ways. These advances include revisions of scales based on new data, the provision of national norms for several assessment instruments, and the coordination of data from multiple informants via cross-informant syndromes scored from parent, teacher, and self-reports. To illuminate the developmental course of empirically based syndromes, we have carried out longitudinal studies that extend into adulthood. Many other studies have now supported the validity and utility of the syndromes.

While empirically based assessment has advanced, health-related services have also undergone major changes since the first edition of this book. The changes reflect the increasing dominance of managed care models, which are imposing new demands on service providers. Empirically based assessment is especially well-suited to meeting managed care demands for standardized documentation of initial problems and for testing outcomes, as well as for comparing the cost-effectiveness of various interventions.

This book presents applications of the empirically based assessment procedures that we have developed. Procedures developed by others will be discussed where relevant, but a survey of such procedures is beyond the scope of this book. Chapter 1 of the book introduces the principles, methods, and goals of empirically based assessment, while Chapter 2 outlines strategies for using empirically based assessment data from multiple sources. Chapter 3 presents research findings on the nature and correlates of empirically based syndromes. In preparation for case illustrations of empirically based assessment, Chapter 4 provides an overview of how the procedures are used in various contexts. Applications to specific cases are illustrated in Chapters 5 through 7, followed in Chapter 8 by a review and integration of the essential features of our approach. All names and personal identifying information in the case material have been changed to protect confidentiality.

Both the development of our empirically based approach and its embodiment in this book owe much to the help of others. For its support of our research on the developmental course of psychopathology, we are especially grateful to the William T. Grant Foundation. Drafts of this book have benefited greatly from critiques by Drs. Bruce Compas and James Hudziak of the University of Vermont, Dr. Michael Epstein of Northern Illinois University, and Dr. Frank Verhulst of Erasmus University, Rotterdam, the Netherlands. For assisting in our recent research, we are grateful to Neil Aguiar, Judith Amour, Janet Arnold, Catherine Howell, David Jacobowitz, Peter Liu, Virginia MacDonald, Catherine Stanger, and Andrew Weine. We deeply appreciate Rachel Berube's diligent work on successive drafts of the manuscript. And, once again, our thanks to Dr. Alan Kazdin, who continues to maintain his superlative record as editor, as well as master of an amazing array of other difficult enterprises.

1

PRINCIPLES, METHODS, AND GOALS OF EMPIRICALLY BASED ASSESSMENT

People who work with troubled children and youths face increasing challenges. On the one hand, public funds for educational and mental health services are being curtailed. On the other hand, there is evidence that behavioral and emotional problems are worsening (Achenbach & Howell, 1993; Johnston, O'Malley, & Bachman, 1995). Family and community resources for supporting healthy development have also eroded, leaving more children without adequate adult supervision.

While the needs for help are growing, changes in systems of care confront practitioners with additional challenges. A particularly pervasive challenge is the shift away from traditional fee-for-service models and toward various managed care models. To meet the challenges of managed care, those who deal with behavioral and emotional problems must maximize the efficacy of their efforts while minimizing costs.

The empirically based approach that we present in this book is designed to facilitate cost-effective assessment, planning, intervention, and outcome evaluation in health, education, and other services that deal with maladaptive behavior among the young. It includes innovative methods for coordinating data from multiple sources in order to provide a comprehensive picture of competencies and problems. We focus mainly on ages 2 to 18, for which we use the term *children* for purposes of brevity. However, we will also touch on applications of our empirically based approach to adults.

This book presents the principles, methods, goals, and applications of our approach, although we will also discuss procedures developed by others where relevant. To illustrate practical applications, we will provide excerpts of cases in which empirically based procedures were used. The case of 12-year-old Kyle provides an introduction to empirically based procedures.

CASE 1: KYLE

At the urging of Kyle's sixth-grade teachers, Kyle's mother sought help for dealing with his behavior. Kyle's teachers reported that he was disruptive and noncompliant and had difficulty getting along with other children. He was also restless and easily distracted in class. In the previous month, Kyle had received detentions at least once a week for fighting or violating school rules. He had a history of behavior problems in kindergarten and first grade, but he had improved in second and third grade. As Kyle approached adolescence, his school problems seemed to escalate. At home, Kyle's problems seemed different from those reported by his teachers. He frequently argued with his parents about homework and household rules, but he was not openly defiant. On some days, he was sullen and had little to do with family members or friends. He also became angry and hostile for no apparent reason. On other days, Kyle was pleasant, cooperative, and fun to be with. Kyle's mother had little idea what produced good or bad days and did not know how to cope with his fluctuating moods and behavior.

Kyle's biological parents had divorced when he was 3 years old, and his mother remarried when he was 5. As part of his stepfather's employee benefit package, the family was enrolled in a health maintenance organization (HMO) where a pediatrician was the primary care provider for Kyle and his two half-sisters. Kyle's mother relied on the pediatrician for advice about behavior management as well as health care for the children. The pediatrician had been particularly helpful in dealing with Kyle's behavior problems when he entered first grade. When Kyle's sixth-grade teachers urged her to seek an evaluation, Kyle's mother made an appointment to see the pediatrician. A physical exam indicated normal development and no medical problems. As part of his evaluation, the pediatrician asked Kyle's mother to complete a standardized form for rating behavioral and emotional problems. The profile scored from the form revealed moderately high scores for attention problems, but higher scores for other kinds of problems. In view of the severity and complexity of the problems revealed by the profile, the pediatrician referred the family to the HMO's mental health service for a comprehensive evaluation.

In assessing Kyle, an HMO psychologist used the data obtained by the pediatrician, plus additional data gathered from Kyle's medical and school records, an interview with his mother, ratings by his stepfather, teacher reports, and direct assessment of Kyle. We focus on the findings obtained with each assessment procedure as we introduce the procedures in this chapter and Chapter 2.

PRINCIPLES OF EMPIRICALLY BASED ASSESSMENT

The principles of empirically based assessment derive partly from psychometric concepts. This means that assessment of behavioral and emotional functioning is viewed as a measurement process that identifies quantitative gradations in the target phenomena. The measurement perspective highlights certain issues that affect all approaches to assessment, as discussed in the following sections.

Measurement Error

All assessment procedures are subject to error. For example, if questions in a structured diagnostic interview are misstated or omitted, or if subjects' responses are incorrectly interpreted or recorded, the diagnoses obtained are likely to differ from those obtained when such mistakes are not made.

Even when no mistakes are made, assessment results are affected by variations in the phenomena being assessed and by variations in the procedures themselves. For example, in structured diagnostic interviews, subjects may initially answer yes to questions about particular symptoms because they carefully search their memories for any hint of such symptoms. However, if the subjects are interviewed again a week later, they often answer no to the same questions. One reason for changing from yes to no may be a subject's decision that the remembered symptom was too trivial to warrant reporting. Another reason may be that subjects wish to avoid the questioning that follows yes answers. A third reason may be that subjects become more impatient with the interview process.

Whatever the reason for changes from affirmative responses in an initial interview to negative responses in a subsequent interview, declines have often been found in symptoms reported by both children (e.g., Edelbrock, Costello, Dulcan, Kalas, & Conover, 1985; Jensen et al., 1995) and adults (e.g., Helzer, Spitznagel, & McEvoy, 1987; Robins, 1985; Vandiver & Sher, 1991). Called the *test-retest attenuation effect,* the tendency to report fewer symptoms in repetitions of an interview produces a significant decline in the number of diagnoses obtained. Even though structured diagnostic interviews are intended to tell us whether a disorder is either present or absent, the results are subject to variations related to the interview process itself.

Variations that are inherent in assessment processes are included in the general term *measurement error,* which also includes variations in the phenomena being assessed and mistakes in applying assessment procedures. Because all assessment procedures are subject to measurement error (i.e., variation), we need ways to deal with variations in the data obtained on every child whom we assess.

Psychometric Guidelines

The psychometric approach is designed to cope with the inevitable variations in assessment data. As applied to our empirically based paradigm, the psychometric approach provides the following guidelines:

1. To minimize error arising from procedural variations, assessment should employ standardized procedures.
2. To avoid error arising from the idiosyncrasies of individual items, multiple items should be used to sample each aspect of functioning.
3. To provide quantitative scores for each aspect of functioning, items should be aggregated into scales.
4. To indicate how individual children compare with relevant reference groups, scores should be normed.
5. For variables related to development, the normative reference groups should be formed according to developmental indices such as age.
6. To be considered psychometrically sound, assessment procedures must be reliable and valid, although the types of reliability and validity vary with the type of procedure.

What Should We Measure?

These six psychometric guidelines, plus a large body of psychometric theory (e.g., Nunnally & Bernstein, 1994), provide standards for sound assessment. However, psychometrics does not dictate what we should measure. In fact, a major challenge for the study of child psychopathology is to identify targets for assessment that will improve our ability to understand, prevent, and treat maladaptive behavior.

One approach to identifying assessment targets is exemplified by the fourth edition of the American Psychiatric Association's (1994) *Diagnostic and Statistical Manual of Mental Disorders (DSM-IV)* and the World Health Organization's (1992) *International Classification of Diseases (ICD)*. The *DSM-IV* and *ICD* diagnostic categories for child psychopathology have been developed largely through negotiations among panels of experts who selected the target disorders and the criteria for defining them. Drafts of the *DSM-IV* categories were also modified on the basis of field trials (McBurnett, Lahey, & Pfiffner, 1993). This approach can be described as working "from the top down," because it starts from decisions about which disorders exist and about how to identify individuals who have each disorder. The dominant approach to assessing such disorders is by interviewing children and their parents about the presence of the criterial features used to define each diagnostic category. The result is a decision about whether a child does or does not have the disorder defined by a particular diagnostic category.

The empirically based approach, by contrast, works "from the ground up." That is, it starts with data on numerous items that describe particular behavioral and emotional problems. Each item is scored on a quantitative scale, such as 0 = *not true of the child,* 1 = *somewhat or sometimes true,* and 2 = *very true or often true.* The ratings are based on a specified period, such as 6 months. Informants such as parents, teachers, and the children themselves use standardized forms on which to rate the items. Multivariate statistical analyses, such as factor analysis and principal components analysis, are then applied to the scores on the problem items to identify sets of problems that tend to occur together. These co-occurring problems make up syndromes in the literal sense of "things that go together." (In its original Greek meaning, *syndrome* referred to the act of running together; Gove, 1971.) Instead of being judged as present versus absent, each syndrome is quantified by summing the scores of the items that compose the syndrome. The result is a syndrome score that reflects the degree to which a child manifests the features of the syndrome.

The empirical identification of syndromes does not involve any assumptions about the causes or course of particular syndromes, nor about whether the syndromes reflect diagnostic categories like those of the *DSM* and *ICD*. Instead, the syndromes provide empirically based starting points for investigating how best to understand the patterns formed by behavioral/emotional problems, as reported by various informants. Because similar standardized rating forms are applicable to children assessed in many contexts, the problem patterns manifested by individual children can be matched to the syndrome patterns that were previously identified in large clinical samples. The syndromes thus serve as focal points for the assessment of individual children, communication about them, the targeting of interventions, and evaluation of outcomes. The syndromes also serve as focal points for research on the causes, correlates, prevention, and treatment of children's behavioral/emotional problems, as detailed in Chapter 3.

Summary of Principles

The main principles of our empirically based paradigm can be summarized as follows:

1. It uses standardized procedures to assess competencies and problems reported by different informants for large samples of children from the target population.
2. The assessment data are analyzed quantitatively to detect associations among problems reported for the samples of children.
3. Syndromes are derived from the identified associations among problems.
4. Scales for scoring individual children are constructed from the items forming the syndromes.
5. Each scale is normed from data on large samples of children, as assessed by particular kinds of informants.
6. Individual children can be evaluated via the same assessment procedures that were used to derive and operationally define the syndromes.

METHODS OF EMPIRICALLY
BASED ASSESSMENT

How are the principles of empirically based assessment used in practice? To implement empirically based assessment, we have developed a family of instruments for obtaining data from parents, teachers, interviewers, observers, and the subjects themselves. For each source of data, we started with a pool of candidate items for rating behavioral/emotional problems. For some instruments, we have also included items for assessing competencies. The candidate items were extensively pilot-tested by having the relevant types of informants complete them for numerous subjects. Successive revisions of the instruments were made to clarify

TABLE 1.1 Construction of Empirically Based Assessment Instruments

1. Write items for intended subjects and informants
2. Test and revise successive editions of items on the basis of feedback from respondents
3. Score large clinical samples of subjects
4. Apply factor analysis or principal components analysis to item scores
5. Identify robust syndromes of co-occurring problems
6. Construct scales for scoring syndromes
7. Obtain normative data for scales
8. Construct scoring profiles

item wording, to add items suggested by the informants, and to delete items that were ineffective.

When the rating instruments and procedures were satisfactory, they were used to score children who had been referred for mental health or special education services. The competence items were tested for their ability to discriminate between referred and nonreferred children. The scores obtained on the problem items were subjected to factor analyses or principal components analyses, which are statistical procedures for identifying sets of problems that tend to co-occur. Multiple procedures were used to detect syndromes of items that repeatedly co-occurred across variations in the statistical analyses. Each syndrome of co-occurring items was then used to construct a scale for scoring that syndrome. Table 1.1 outlines the sequence of steps involved in developing the empirically based assessment instruments. Using the sequence outlined in Table 1.1, we have developed instruments for obtaining ratings of children, adolescents, and young adults from multiple informants under various conditions.

The Child Behavior Checklist for Ages 4 to 18

To illustrate the sequence outlined in Table 1.1, we will use the Child Behavior Checklist for Ages 4-18 (CBCL/4-18), which obtains reports of children's competencies and problems from parents and parent surrogates. Pages 1 and 2 of the CBCL/4-18 display questions about the amount and quality of the child's participation in sports, nonsports activities, organizations, jobs and chores, friendships, relationships with significant others; the manner in which the child plays and works alone; and the child's school performance. There are also open-ended questions about any disabilities the child has, what concerns the parent most about the child, and the best things about the child.

Pages 3 and 4 of the CBCL/4-18 display descriptions of 118 behavioral/emotional problems, such as *Acts too young for age, Cries a lot, Cruel to animals, Sets fires,* and *Unhappy, sad, or depressed.* Open-ended items are also provided for the respondent to add physical problems without known medical cause and other problems that are not specifically described on the CBCL. For each item, the respondent is asked to circle 0 if it is not true of the child, 1 if it is somewhat or sometimes true, and 2 if it is very true or often true, based on the preceding 6 months.

Scales for Scoring the CBCL Competence Items. The competence items are scored on three scales designated as Activities, Social, and School. Figure 1.1 illustrates a hand-scored version of the profile for displaying the competence scales. The profile shown in Figure 1.1 was scored from the CBCL/4-18 completed by the mother of Kyle, the boy who was introduced at the beginning of this chapter. Scores for each item of the Activities scale are summed to yield a total score for Activities, which is entered beneath the items composing the scale. The same procedure is followed to compute the scores for the Social and School scales, which are displayed to the right of the Activities scale in Figure 1.1.

To draw a profile in the graphic display above the scales, the user marks the total score for each scale in the column of numbers above the scale. The user then draws lines to connect the scores that have been marked for the three scales, as illustrated in Figure 1.1. To help the user compare Kyle's scores on the competence scales with the scores of normal peers, the left side of the profile displays percentiles for scores obtained by a national sample of boys who had not been referred for mental health services during the preceding 12 months. Compared to this normative sample, Kyle's score on the Activities scale corresponded to the 31st percentile, his score on the Social scale corresponded to the 2nd percentile, and his score on the School scale corresponded to the 5th percentile.

The broken lines printed on the profile at the 2nd and 5th percentiles demarcate a borderline clinical range. Beneath the lower broken lines are exceptionally low scores that are considered to be in the clinical range because they are lower than the scores obtained by 98% of boys in the normative sample. Above the upper broken line are scores that are in the normal range because they are higher than the lowest 5% of scores in the normative sample. As Figure 1.1 shows, Kyle's score on the Activities scale was in the normal range, whereas his scores on the Social and School

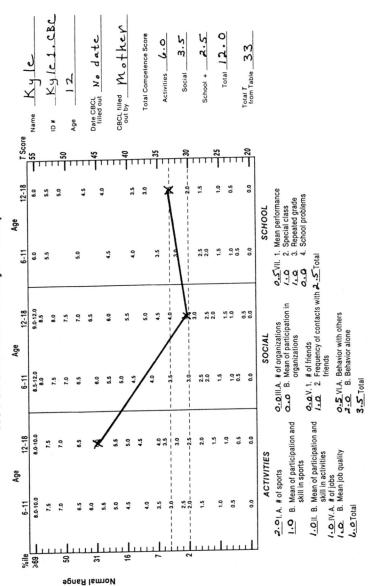

Figure 1.1. Hand-scored CBCL competence profile for 12-year-old Kyle.

scales were in the borderline clinical range. Kyle's high score on the Activities scale reflected his mother's positive reports about his involvement in sports, hobbies, free-time activities, and chores at home. Compared to other children of the same age, Kyle's mother rated him average to above average in several sports and average in activities and job quality. Kyle's lower scores on the Social and School scales reflected the fact that he was not involved in any social organizations, had few friends, and had poor grades in several academic subjects. In addition to the percentiles displayed on the left side of the profile, T scores are displayed on the right side to provide a common numerical scale whereby a particular T score has a similar meaning for all three competence scales.

Scales for Scoring the CBCL Problem Items. In addition to hand-scoring of the CBCL profile, the profile can also be scored by a computer program. A computer-scored version of the problem scales of Kyle's profile is shown in Figure 1.2. The profile displays eight syndromes that were derived from statistical analyses of problems scored on the CBCL/4-18 for 4,455 children who had been referred for mental health services. (The analyses were principal components analyses, with varimax rotations, as detailed by Achenbach, 1991b.) The derivation of syndromes from parents' ratings was coordinated with analyses of teacher- and self-ratings in order to identify patterns of problems that had counterparts in multiple sources of data, as explained in Chapter 2.

The profile shown in Figure 1.2 displays the scores (0, 1, or 2) that Kyle received for each problem item on the CBCL completed by his mother. Like the competence scales that were shown in Figure 1.1, the syndrome scales are scored by summing the scores of the items that compose each syndrome. The computer program prints the raw score obtained on each syndrome at the bottom of the syndrome scale. The program also prints a mark in the graphic display above the syndrome scale to show where the child's score is located in relation to the scores obtained by the normative sample of peers. As shown in Figure 1.2, Kyle's raw score on the leftmost syndrome, designated as Withdrawn, was 6, which is at the 93rd percentile of the normative sample. Note that high scores, indicating relatively numerous problems, are clinically important on this portion of the profile. (On the competence portion of the profile, low scores are clinically important, because they indicate a lack of competence.) After the program has printed out the profile, the user can draw lines to connect the marked scores in the graphic display, if desired.

The broken lines printed on the profile in Figure 1.2 demarcate a borderline clinical range from the 95th to the 98th percentiles of the normative sample (*T* scores from 67 to 70). Scores below the lower broken line are considered to be in the normal range, because they are below the 95th percentile. Scores above the upper broken line are considered to be in the clinical range, because they indicate more problems than were reported for 98% of the normative sample. As Figure 1.2 shows, Kyle's scores on the Thought Problems and Aggressive Behavior syndromes were in the clinical range (above the 98th percentile), whereas his score on the Delinquent Behavior syndrome was in the borderline range, and his scores on the other syndromes were in the normal range.

Beneath each syndrome scale, the computer program prints out a *T* score that compares the child's syndrome score with scores from the normative sample of nonreferred peers, plus a second *T* score that compares the child's syndrome score with scores from a large sample of children referred for mental health services (Achenbach, 1993, provides details of these clinical *T* scores). In addition to the syndromes, the problem portion of the profile also displays scores for problem items that are on the CBCL but that are not consistently enough associated with any one syndrome to be included in a syndrome scale. Scores for these items, plus a total problem score and scores for Internalizing and Externalizing groupings of syndromes, are displayed to the right of the profile, as shown in Figure 1.2.

A single + sign is printed beside any Internalizing, Externalizing, or total problem score that is in the borderline clinical range. Two + signs are printed beside any of these scores that are in the clinical range, as shown on the upper right side of Kyle's profile in Figure 1.2. The borderline range on the Internalizing, Externalizing, and total problem scores extends from the 82nd to the 90th percentile (*T* scores from 60 to 63). Scores below the 82nd percentile are in the normal range, whereas scores above the 90th percentile are in the clinical range. Note that the borderline and clinical ranges start at lower percentiles on the Internalizing, Externalizing, and total problem scales than on the syndrome scales, where the borderline range starts at the 95th percentile and the clinical range starts above the 98th percentile. The reason for defining the borderline and clinical ranges in terms of higher percentiles on the syndrome scales is that each syndrome scale has fewer items and covers a narrower domain than the Internalizing, Externalizing, and total problem scales. (The higher cutpoints on the syndrome scales are designed to avoid higher rates of false positives that could result from the narrower sampling of

12

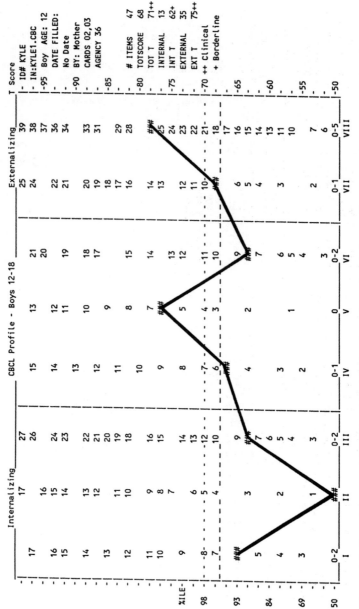

Figure 1.2. Computer-scored CBCL problem profile for 12-year-old Kyle.

WITHDRAWN	SOMATIC COMPLAINTS	ANXIOUS/ DEPRESSED	SOCIAL PROBLEMS	THOUGHT PROBLEMS	ATTENTION PROBLEMS	DELINQUENT BEHAVIOR	AGGRESSIVE BEHAVIOR	OTHER PROBS
2 42.Rather-BeAlone	0 51. Dizzy	0 12.Lonely	0 1. Acts Young	2 9. Mind Off	0 1. Acts Young	1 26.NoGuilt	2 3. Argues	0 5. ActOppSex
1 65.Won't Talk	0 54. Tired	0 14.Cries	2 11.Clings	0 40.Hears Things	1 8. Concen-trate	2 39.BadCompan	2 7. Brags	0 6. BM Out
1 69.Secret-ive	0 56a.Aches	0 31.FearDoBad	2 25.NotGet Along	2 66.Repeats Acts	2 10.Sit Still	2 43.LieCheat	1 16.Mean	0 15.CruelAnim
0 75.Shy	0 56b.Head-aches	0 32.Perfect	2 38.Teased	0 70.Sees Acts	0 13.Confuse	0 63.PrefOlder	0 19.DemAttn	0 18.HarmSelf
0 80.Stares	0 56c.Nausea	1 33.Unloved	2 48.Not Liked	0 70.Sees Things	0 17.Day-dream	0 67.RunAway	0 20.DestOwn	0 24.NotEat
1 88.Sulks	0 56d.Eye	2 34.OutToGet	0 55.Over-Weight*	0 80.Stares*	2 41.Impulsv	0 72.SetFires	0 21 DestOthr	0 28.EatNonFood
0 102.Under-active	0 56e.Skin	1 35.Worthless	0 62.Clumsy	1 84.Strange Behav	2 45.Nervous	1 81.StealHome	2 22.DisbHome*	0 29.Fears
1 103.Sad	0 56f.Stomach	2 45.Nervous	0 64.Prefers Young	1 85.Strange Ideas	0 46.Twitch*	1 82.StealOut	2 23.DisbSchl	0 30.FearSchool
0 111.With-drawn	0 56g.Vomit	0 50.Fearful			1 61.Poor School	1 90.Swears	1 27.Jealous	0 36.GetHurt
		0 52.Guilty				0 96.ThinkSex*	2 37.Fights	0 44.BiteNail
		0 71.SelfConsc				0 101.Truant	1 57.Attacks	0 47.Nightmares
		1 89.Suspic				0 105.AlcDrugs	1 68.Screams	0 49.Constipate
		1 103.Sad				0 106.Vandal*	2 74.ShowOff	0 53.Overeat
		0 112.Worries					2 86.Stubborn	0 56h.OtherPhys
							1 87.MoodChng	0 58.PickSkin
							1 93.TalkMuch	0 59.SexPrtsP
							1 94.Teases	0 60.SexPrtsM
							2 95.Temper	0 73.SexProbs
							2 97.Threaten	0 76.SleepLess
							2 104.Loud	0 77.SleepMore
6 TOTAL	0 TOTAL	8 TOTAL	5 TOTAL	6 TOTAL	8 TOTAL	8 TOTAL	27 TOTAL	0 78.SmearBM
65 T SCORE	50 T SCORE	63 T SCORE	66 T SCORE	76 T SCORE	63 T SCORE	68 T SCORE	79 T SCORE	0 79.SpeechProb
50 CLIN T	41 CLIN T	47 CLIN T	50 CLIN T	66 CLIN T	46 CLIN T	52 CLIN T	62 CLIN T	1 83.StoresUp
								1 91.TalkSuicid
								0 92.SleepWalk
								0 98.ThumbSuck
								0 99.TooNeat
								0 100.SleepProb
								0 107.WetsSelf
								0 108.WetsBed
								0 109.Whining
								0 110.WshOpSex
								1 113.OtherProb

*Items not on Cross-Informant Construct

Not in Total Problem Score
0 2.Allergy 0 4.Asthma

Profile Type:	WTHDR	SOMAT	SOCIAL	DEL-AGG	W-A/D-Agg	Soc-Att	Delinq
ICC:	-.179	-.510	.270	.317	.125	.011	-.036

No ICCs are significant

Figure 1.2. (Continued)

13

TABLE 1.2 Empirically Based Assessment Instruments

Instruments	Informants	Subjects' Ages	References
Child Behavior Checklist for Ages 2-3 (CBCL/2-3)	Parents	2 to 3	Achenbach, 1992b
Teacher/Caregiver Report Form for Ages 2-5 (TCRF/2-5)	Teachers, day care providers	2 to 5	Achenbach, 1995
Child Behavior Checklist for Ages 4-18 (CBCL/4-18)	Parents	4 to 18	Achenbach, 1991b
Teacher's Report Form (TRF)	Teachers	5 to 18	Achenbach, 1991c
Youth Self-Report (YSR)	Youths	11 to 18	Achenbach, 1991d
Young Adult Behavior Checklist (YABCL)	Parents	19 to 30	Achenbach et al., 1995c
Young Adult Self-Report (YASR)	Young adults	19 to 30	Achenbach et al., 1995c
Semistructured Clinical Interview for Children and Adolescents (SCICA)	Interviewers	6 to 18	McConaughy & Achenbach, 1994b
Direct Observation Form (DOF)	Observers of behavior in group settings	5 to 14	Achenbach, 1991b

problems on each syndrome scale than on the Internalizing, Externalizing, and total problem scales.)

In addition to the CBCL/4-18 for obtaining parents' ratings, our other empirically based assessment instruments are listed in Table 1.2, with the intended informants, the subjects' age ranges, and the primary publication reference for each one. These instruments will be described further in Chapter 2.

GOALS OF EMPIRICALLY
BASED ASSESSMENT

Our empirically based paradigm is intended to improve understanding of adaptive and maladaptive development and to improve our ways of facilitating development through research, prevention, treatment, and education. Empirically based assessment is fully compatible with other paradigms, such as those embodied in the *DSM, ICD,* behavioral, pharmacological, genetic, neuropsychiatric, educational, family, and psychodynamic approaches. Each of these approaches may have special relevance for particular contexts and particular practitioners. However, the empirically based paradigm provides a common descriptive language for behavioral and emotional functioning that can be used in conjunction with these other approaches to attain the goals presented in the following sections.

Low-Cost Assessment

Initial assessment data can be obtained by having parents, teachers, and youths independently complete standardized forms in 15 to 20 minutes, at no cost in professional time. Clerical workers can hand-score or computer-score the data. Options are also available for using machine-scorable forms and direct computer entry of data by parents, teachers, and youths. Mental health, special education, and health care personnel can readily assimilate the data, which are displayed in profile formats. Related procedures are applicable to clinical interviews and to direct observations in group settings, such as classrooms.

Diverse Users and Purposes

By making it easy for users from diverse backgrounds to routinely obtain similar standardized data, the empirically based approach facilitates communication among different professions. The documentation of competencies and problems via reports by various informants also provides explicit targets for intervention. Because the competencies and problems are quantified and the assessment procedures can be periodically readministered, users can measure changes from the initial baseline assessment to subsequent reassessments. Furthermore, as recommended by Jacobson and Truax (1991), the norms enable users to judge the clinical significance of intervention effects. That is, because the norms indicate the degree of deviance, users can judge whether pre- to post-intervention changes are clinically important, according to whether scores move from the clinical to the normal range.

Application of Knowledge
From Previous Cases

In addition to improving assessment of individual children, the empirically based paradigm is intended to assist users in applying knowledge gained through previous research and clinical experience to new cases. For example, suppose that children who have scores elevated on a particular syndrome have been found to benefit from Treatment A more than Treatment B. New cases that are elevated on this syndrome are therefore apt to be better candidates for Treatment A than B. Another way of applying empirically based findings is to identify the distinguishing characteristics of children who typically have poor outcomes. If children having particular patterns of scores are found to have poor outcomes, we should develop innovative interventions for new cases whose intake assessments yield patterns like those that have been found to predict poor outcomes.

Advancement of Training

A further goal of empirically based assessment is to advance the training of practitioners and researchers. If trainees can quickly obtain standardized data from informants on all cases, they will have more time to customize the aspects of assessment that are not so easily standardized. For example, when trainees have learned to identify areas of deviance and nondeviance in the standardized data, they can begin focusing their interview efforts on building rapport with children and parents, obtaining information to illuminate areas of deviance, and exploring inconsistencies between reports by different informants. Under managed care, it is especially important to maximize the cost-effectiveness of expensive procedures, such as clinical interviews.

To ensure that trainees have adequate experience with different kinds of problems, supervisors can use empirically based assessment to select cases whose syndrome scores show deviance in the areas targeted for training. To sharpen trainees' assessment skills, they can complete the same standardized rating forms that are completed by parents or other informants and can conduct empirically based interviews. Comparisons between the trainees' data and data from the other informants can then be made at different points in services to help the trainees become aware of possible differences among informants' reports of changes.

Summary of Goals

Practical ways to achieve the goals of empirically based assessment will be illustrated throughout the book. In the meantime, the main goals can be summarized as follows:

1. To facilitate healthy behavioral and emotional development through research, prevention, treatment, and education.

2. To provide a common descriptive language for behavioral and emotional functioning that can be used in conjunction with other approaches, such as the *DSM* and *ICD* approaches.

3. To make it easy and economical for users from diverse backgrounds to routinely obtain similar standardized data.

4. To facilitate communication among practitioners from different professions.

5. To enable users to measure changes in functioning from initial baseline assessments to subsequent reassessments.

6. To enable users to judge the clinical significance of changes by determining whether scores have moved from the clinical range to the normal range.

7. To assist users in applying knowledge gained from previous cases to new cases.

8. To advance the training of practitioners and researchers by freeing them to customize the aspects of assessment that cannot be standardized.

9. To identify cases manifesting the different kinds of deviance that trainees should learn about.

10. To sharpen trainees' assessment skills by having them complete the standardized assessment forms and empirically based interviews for comparison with data obtained from other sources.

In Chapter 2, we outline strategies for using empirically based assessment data from multiple sources. Chapter 3 presents research findings related to particular empirically based syndromes, and Chapter 4 shows how empirically based procedures are applied in various contexts. Practical applications to specific cases are illustrated in Chapters 5 through 7. In Chapter 8, we review and integrate the applications of empirically based assessment.

SUMMARY

The empirically based paradigm is designed to facilitate cost-effective planning and accountability in health, education, and other services dealing with maladaptive behavior.

Assessment of behavioral and emotional functioning is viewed as a measurement process that identifies quantitative gradations in the target phenomena and that provides a basis for determining which characteristics co-occur to form syndromes. All assessment procedures are subject to variations (measurement error) that must be considered in drawing conclusions about behavioral and emotional functioning.

The principles of empirically based assessment include psychometric standards for the quality of assessment procedures, plus the use of standardized procedures, large samples of subjects, and quantitative analyses to construct normed scales with which to assess new cases.

Empirically based assessment provides a descriptive language for behavioral and emotional functioning that can be used in conjunction with many other approaches to advance research, prevention, treatment, and education. It employs standardized forms for obtaining quantified reports from parents, teachers, interviewers, observers, and the children themselves. The data are scored on profiles of scales that enable users to compare individual children with reference samples of peers.

The goals of empirically based assessment include (a) providing easy and economical assessment by diverse users; (b) facilitating use of practical clinical data by researchers, the use of research findings by practitioners, and communication about cases; (c) enabling users to measure changes in reported competencies and problems and to judge the clinical significance of the changes; (d) assisting users in applying knowledge gained from previous cases to new cases; and (e) advancing the training of practitioners and researchers.

2

STRATEGIES FOR USING EMPIRICALLY BASED ASSESSMENT

In Chapter 1, we introduced the principles, methods, and goals of empirically based assessment. In this chapter, we outline strategies for using empirically based assessment data from multiple sources. As Chapter 1 emphasized, empirically based assessment is designed to cope with the variations that affect all assessment procedures. In addition to the variations that affect each assessment procedure unto itself, the assessment of behavioral and emotional functioning must cope with the variations among different sources of information.

Children's functioning often varies from one context and interaction partner to another. Furthermore, the informants themselves may contribute additional variation, owing to differences in what they notice, their standards for judging children, and their candor. Situational variations in children's behavior and variations between informants both may limit the agreement found between reports by different informants. The typical levels of agreement between informants are indicated by the following correlations found by averaging the results of studies that used many different assessment instruments: Between informants who play similar roles in relation to the children they judge (e.g., pairs of parents; pairs of teachers), the mean correlation was .60; between pairs of informants who play different roles in relation to the children (e.g., parents versus teachers), the mean correlation was .28; and between children's self-reports and reports by others (parents, teachers, mental health workers), the mean correlation was .22 (Achenbach, McConaughy, & Howell, 1987). Although modest, all these cross-informant correlations were statistically significant. It is therefore clear that reports by different informants do capture certain cross-situational consistencies in children's functioning. However, it is equally clear that what one informant reports about a child is apt to differ in some respects from what other informants report about the same child.

MULTIAXIAL ASSESSMENT

Because agreement among informants is far from perfect, no one informant can substitute for all others. Instead, each informant can convey a picture of the child's functioning in a particular context, as seen from that informant's perspective. When the informants are significant figures in the child's life, such as parents, teachers, and mental health workers, their perspectives are key ingredients in the evaluation of the child.

In addition to reports by informants, other kinds of data are also relevant to the assessment of most children. These include medical data and standardized tests of ability and achievement. Together, the multiple sources and kinds of data compose a model for multiaxial assessment that can guide practitioners' thinking, their choice of procedures, and the decisions they need to make about how to help children. Table 2.1 summarizes multiaxial assessment in terms of five axes designated as Parent Reports, Teacher Reports, Cognitive Assessment, Physical Assessment, and Direct Assessment of the Child, which includes interviews, observations, and self-reports.

Not all axes or procedures shown in Table 2.1 are relevant to all cases. For example, Axis 2, Teacher Reports, would not be relevant for children who do not attend school. On the other hand, additional axes might also be considered, such as assessment of family functioning via procedures that vary according to the diverse family constellations in which today's children live. We will focus mainly on the empirically based assessment procedures that we have developed for parent reports, teacher reports, and direct assessment of the child. However, procedures developed by others will be discussed in the context of case examples.

The multiaxial model provides a strategic framework for organizing assessment concepts, plans, and procedures. It emphasizes standardized and reliable procedures for obtaining multisource assessment data about each case. Of the empirically based instruments for assessing behavioral and emotional problems listed in Table 2.1, the CBCL/4-18 was introduced in Chapter 1. The Teacher's Report Form (TRF) and Youth Self-Report (YSR) are parallel instruments for obtaining teacher and self-ratings of

TABLE 2.1 Examples of Multiaxial Assessment Procedures

Age Range	*Axis I* *Parent Reports*	*Axis II* *Teacher Reports*	*Axis III* *Cognitive Assessment*	*Axis IV* *Physical Assessment*	*Axis V* *Direct Assessment* *of Child*
2 to 5	CBCL/2-3 CBCL/4-18 Developmental history Parent interview Vineland Social Maturity Scale (Sparrow et al., 1984)	TCRF/2-5 Preschool record Teacher interview	Ability tests, e.g., McCarthy (1972) Perceptual-motor tests Language tests	Height, weight Medical exam Neurological exam	Observation during testing and play interview
6 to 11	CBCL/4-18 Developmental history Parent interview	TRF School records Teacher interview	Ability tests, e.g., Kaufman & Kaufman (1983) Achievement tests Perceptual-motor tests Language tests	Height, weight Medical exam Neurological exam	SCICA DOF
12 to 18	CBCL/4-18 Developmental history Parent interview	TRF School records Teacher interview	Ability tests, e.g., WAIS-R; WISC-III, (Wechsler, 1981, 1991) Achievement tests	Height, weight Medical exam Neurological exam	SCICA DOF YSR Self-concept measures Personality tests

NOTE: Unfamiliar acronyms can be found in the List of Acronyms at the front of this book.

many of the same problem items rated by parents on the CBCL/4-18, but the wording of the items is adapted for teachers and 11- to 18-year-old youths, respectively.

On the TRF, 25 CBCL/4-18 problem items that most teachers would not be able to rate (e.g., *Nightmares*) are replaced by items that teachers are especially knowledgeable about (e.g., *Disrupts class discipline*). To allow time for teachers to rate children at multiple points throughout the school year, the baseline period for rating TRF problems is 2 months, rather than the 6 months specified on the CBCL/4-18. Furthermore, because teachers are not usually able to report details of the CBCL/4-18 activities and social competence items, the TRF instead requests ratings of the following aspects of school-related adaptive functioning: how hard the child is working; how appropriately the child is behaving; how much the child is learning; and how happy the child is. Teachers are also asked to rate the child's performance in each academic subject on 5-point scales that range from *far below grade* to *far above grade*.

On the YSR, 16 of the CBCL/4-18 problem items that are inappropriate for adolescent self-ratings (e.g., *Thumb-sucking*) are replaced with socially desirable items (e.g., *I like to help others*), thus leaving 102 problem items. The YSR includes competence items like those on the CBCL/4-18 but does not include items concerning grade repetition and special class placement. The other empirically based assessment instruments listed in Table 2.1 will be discussed in later sections.

By using the CBCL/4-18, TRF, and YSR to obtain initial assessment data with little expenditure of their own time, practitioners can invest more time in tailoring other aspects of assessment to the specific needs of each child. As an example, if exceptionally large discrepancies are found between reports by a child's mother and father, the practitioner can explore the reasons for the discrepancies when interviewing the parents. This can be clinically informative, as it may reveal important differences in the child's behavior with each parent, differences between the behavior of the mother versus father toward the child, or differences between the parents' perceptions of what may in fact be consistent behavior by the child.

If exceptionally large discrepancies are found between reports by different teachers, classroom observations can be used to determine how much the child's behavior varies between classes. If observations confirm major variations in the child's behavior, then the specific effects of particular teachers and classes should be considered in designing interventions. On the other hand, if the child's behavior is not found to vary in the ways implied by the discrepant teacher reports, then certain teachers' perceptions of the child may need changing.

CROSS-INFORMANT SYNDROMES
SCORED FROM THE CBCL/4-18, TRF, AND YSR

Analyses of the CBCL/4-18, TRF, and YSR have identified syndromes of co-occurring problems that have counterparts for both genders and multiple age groups, as seen by different kinds of informants (Achenbach, 1991a). These cross-informant syndromes enable users to compare parent, teacher, and self-ratings for similar patterns of problems. We found eight syndromes that had counterparts in a majority of the gender/age groups, as scored on at least two of the three rating instruments. The eight cross-informant syndromes were given the following labels: Withdrawn, Somatic Complaints, Anxious Depressed, Social Problems, Thought Problems, Attention Problems, Delinquent Behavior, and Aggressive Behavior.

To reflect both the similarities and the differences between patterns derived from different informants, the scales for scoring the syndromes comprise not only items that are common across informants, but also items that are specific to the version of a syndrome that was derived from only one type of informant. For example, our statistical analyses showed that the item *Disrupts class discipline* was included in the version of the Aggressive Behavior syndrome that was derived from the TRF. Because most parents would not be able to observe that their child disrupts class discipline and because youths are unlikely to report it about themselves, it is not included on the CBCL/4-18 or the YSR. It could therefore not be included in the version of the Aggressive Behavior syndrome scored from these instruments. Nevertheless, because it is an important part of the Aggressive Behavior syndrome as seen by teachers, it is included on the Aggressive Behavior syndrome scale scored from the TRF.

Table 2.2 lists the problem items that compose the eight cross-informant syndromes, as they are scored from at least two of the three instruments. Those items that are omitted from one of the instruments are indicated by superscripts in Table 2.2. Additional items that are specific to the scoring of a syndrome from only one instrument—such as *Disrupts class discipline* on the TRF Aggressive Behavior scale—are not shown in Table 2.2 but are displayed on the profile scored from that instrument.

TABLE 2.2 Items Defining the Cross-Informant Syndrome Constructs Derived From the Child Behavior Checklist, Youth Self-Report, and Teacher's Report Form

Internalizing Scales		Neither Internalizing Nor Externalizing		Externalizing Scales	
Withdrawn	*Anxious/Depressed*	*Social Problems*	*Attention Problems*	*Delinquent Behavior*	*Aggressive Behavior*
42. Would rather be alone	12. Lonely	1. Acts too young	1. Acts too young	26. Lacks guilt	3. Argues
65. Refuses to talk	14. Cries a lot	11. Too dependent	8. Can't concentrate	39. Bad companions	7. Brags
69. Secretive	31. Fears impulses	25. Doesn't get along with peers	10. Can't sit still	43. Lies	16. Mean to others
75. Shy, timid	32. Needs to be perfect	38. Gets teased	13. Confused	63. Prefers older kids	19. Demands attention
80. Stares blankly[a]	33. Feels unloved	48. Not liked by peers	17. Daydreams	67. Runs away from home[b]	20. Destroys own things
88. Sulks[a]	34. Feels persecuted	62. Clumsy	41. Impulsive	72. Sets fires[b]	21. Destroys others' things
102. Underactive	35. Feels worthless,	64. Prefers younger kids	45. Nervous, tense	81. Steals at home[b]	23. Disobedient at school
103. Unhappy, sad, depressed	45. Nervous, tense		61. Poor schoolwork	82. Steals outside home	27. Jealous
111. Withdrawn	50. Fearful, anxious		62. Clumsy	90. Swearing, obscenity	37. Fights
	52. Feels too guilty	*Thought Problems*	80. Stares blankly[a]	101. Truancy	57. Attacks people
Somatic Complaints	71. Self-conscious	9. Can't get mind off thoughts		105. Alcohol, drugs	68. Screams
51. Feels dizzy	89. Suspicious	40. Hears things			74. Shows off
54. Overtired	103. Unhappy, sad, depressed	66. Repeats acts			86. Stubborn, sullen
56a. Aches, pains	112. Worries	70. Sees things			87. Sudden moods
56b. Headaches		84. Strange behavior			93. Talks too much
56c. Nausea		85. Strange ideas			94. Teases
56d. Eye problems					95. Temper tantrums
56e. Skin problems					97. Threatens
56f. Stomachaches					104. Loud
56g. Vomiting					

SOURCE: Achenbach (1991a).
NOTE: Items are designated by the numbers they bear on the CBCL, YSR, and TRF and by summaries of their content.
a. Not on YSR.
b. Not on TRF.

Syndromes as Hypothetical Constructs

Each syndrome can be viewed as representing a *hypothetical construct*—that is, a pattern of functioning that is hypothesized or inferred from the sets of problems found to co-occur in the analyses of the CBCL/4-18, TRF, and YSR. For a particular child, the construct for each syndrome can be measured by summing the child's scores obtained from a particular informant on the relevant syndrome scale of the CBCL/4-18, TRF, or YSR. Differences between informants and between some of the items that appear on the CBCL/4-18 versus the TRF versus the YSR, as well as variations in the child's behavior, may contribute to differences among the syndrome scores obtained by a child on the different instruments. The syndrome score that is obtained from a particular informant, such as a score for the Aggressive Behavior syndrome obtained from a teacher, is thus just one of several possible measurements of the syndrome construct for the child. Other possible measurements of the syndrome construct include CBCL ratings by the child's mother and father, YSR ratings by the child, and TRF ratings by other teachers. In statistical terms, the syndrome can also be viewed as a *latent variable*—that is, a variable whose values are inferred from multiple measures.

Gender and Age Variations in Scores

The scales for scoring the syndromes take account of variations in problems that are related to the gender and age of the children who are rated, as well as to differences in the types of informants who rate the children. This is done by providing separate norms, standard scores, and clinical cutpoints for boys versus girls within particular age ranges, as rated by each type of informant.

As an example, on the Aggressive Behavior scale scored from the TRF, the 98th percentile score is 22 for 5- to 11-year-old girls, but is 29 for 5- to 11-year-old boys. This means that, because teachers rate girls considerably lower than boys on Aggressive Behavior, a girl who obtains a score of 22 would be as deviant from most girls as a boy who obtains a score of 29 is deviant from most boys. Because the scores for girls are so much lower than for boys, application of a cutpoint based on boys would miss girls who are quite deviant from most other girls with respect to the Aggressive Behavior syndrome. In parents' ratings, however, the gender difference is considerably smaller, as the 98th percentile score for Aggressive Behavior is 20 for girls versus 22 for boys.

Internalizing and Externalizing
Groupings of Syndromes

In Table 2.2, the Withdrawn, Somatic Complaints, and Anxious/Depressed syndromes are listed under the heading Internalizing; the Social Problems, Thought Problems, and Attention Problems syndromes are listed under the heading Neither Internalizing nor Externalizing; and the Delinquent Behavior and Aggressive Behavior syndromes are listed under the heading Externalizing. The Internalizing and Externalizing groupings reflect associations among syndromes that were identified through second-order factor analyses of correlations among the syndromes (Achenbach, 1991a; a factor analysis is called *second-order* when it is performed on correlations between variables that were themselves derived from *first-order* factor analytic procedures, as the syndromes were). The syndromes that are designated as Neither Internalizing nor Externalizing were not as strongly associated with either the Internalizing or Externalizing groupings as were the syndromes that are included in these groupings. A child's score for Internalizing is obtained by summing the scores of the items on the three Internalizing syndromes, whereas the child's score for Externalizing is obtained by summing the items on the two Externalizing syndromes.

PROFILES FOR DISPLAYING
CROSS-INFORMANT SYNDROME SCALES

To help users compare a child's standing on each syndrome as scored by a particular informant with the child's standing on that syndrome as scored by other informants, the profiles from all three instruments display the eight cross-informant syndromes in the same sequence from left to right. However, the profiles also differ somewhat, in that the specific items displayed for each syndrome scale are just the items that are scored on that scale by the relevant informant.

As an example, the computer-scored TRF profile shown in Figure 2.1 (on pages 28-29) for 12-year-old Kyle lists the items of each syndrome scale that were scored from his math teacher's ratings, whether or not those particular items are included in the CBCL/4-18 versions of the syndromes (which were shown in Figure 1.2) or in the YSR versions of the syndromes. To compare Kyle's TRF syndrome scores with those of a normative sample of peers, his profile displays percentiles (on the left side of the graphic display) and *T* scores (on the right side and beneath each syndrome scale) that are based on scores obtained by a national sample of nonreferred 12- to 18-year-old boys, as rated by their teachers. As Figure 2.1 shows, Kyle's math teacher reported so many problems of the Aggressive Behavior syndrome (the rightmost syndrome on the profile), that his score for this syndrome was well up in the clinical range (T score = 90). The math teacher's TRF also yielded scores in the borderline clinical range on the Anxious/Depressed, Social Problems, and Delinquent Behavior syndromes (scales III, IV, and VII in Figure 2.1).

Cross-Informant Comparisons
of Item and Scale Scores

The similar layouts for the three profiles make it easy for users to compare a child's patterns of syndrome scores by looking at the profiles obtained from parent, teacher, and self-ratings. For example, look at Kyle's TRF profile in Figure 2.1 and then look at Kyle's CBCL profile in Figure 1.2. You can see that Kyle obtained high scores on the Delinquent Behavior and Aggressive Behavior syndromes from both his math teacher and his mother. However, you can also see that the TRF yielded high scores on the Anxious/Depressed and Social Problems syndromes, whereas the CBCL yielded high scores on the Thought Problems syndrome.

To help users make systematic comparisons between multiple raters of the same child (or ratings by the same person on multiple occasions), a cross-informant computer program is available that can score a child's profiles from up to five CBCLs, TRFs, and/or YSRs (Arnold & Jacobowitz, 1993). The program also prints side-by-side displays of the scores obtained from each form. This makes it easy for users to see items and scales on which there is good versus poor agreement among informants.

As an example, Figure 2.2 displays a portion of the side-by-side comparisons between item scores that were obtained for Kyle from ratings by his mother, stepfather, math teacher, and English teacher, as well as from Kyle's self-ratings on the YSR. By looking at Figure 2.2, you can see that on the Withdrawn scale, the topmost item, 42. *Would rather be alone than with others,* was rated as being true of Kyle (scores of 1 or 2) by all informants except Kyle's English teacher. The fourth item down, 75. *Shy,* was rated as not true of Kyle by all five informants. Looking to the right side of Table 2.3, you can see that all five informants rated items 25. *Doesn't get along with other kids* and 38. *Gets teased a lot* as true of Kyle, and all except Kyle himself rated 48. *Not liked by other kids* as true.

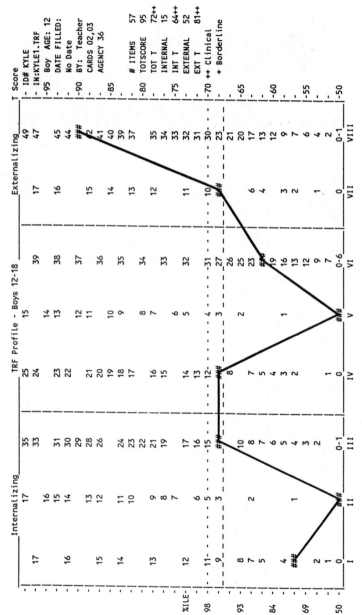

Figure 2.1. TRF Problem Profile for 12-year-old Kyle.

WITHDRAWN
- 1 42.Rather BeAlone
- 0 65.Won't Talk
- 0 69.Secretive
- 0 75.Shy
- 0 80.Stares
- 1 88.Sulks
- 0 102.Underactive
- 0 TOTAL
- 1 103.Sad
- 0 111.Withdrawn
- 3 TOTAL
- 57 T SCORE
- 44 CLIN T

SOMATIC COMPLAINTS
- 0 51. Dizzy
- 0 54. Tired
- 0 56a.Aches
- 0 56b.Head-aches
- 0 56c.Nausea
- 0 56d.Eye
- 0 56e.Skin
- 0 56f.Stomach
- 0 56g.Vomit
- 0 TOTAL
- 50 T SCORE
- 44 CLIN T

ANXIOUS/DEPRESSED
- 0 12.Lonely
- 1 14.Cries
- 0 31.FearDoBad
- 0 32.Perfect
- 1 33.Unloved
- 2 34.OutoGet
- 0 35.Worthless
- 1 45.Nervous
- 0 47.Conforms*
- 0 50.Fearful
- 0 52.Guilty
- 0 71.SelfConsc
- 2 81.HurtCrit*
- 2 89.Suspic
- 1 103.Sad
- 1 108.Mistake*
- 1 112.Worries
- 13 TOTAL
- 69 T SCORE
- 57 CLIN T

SOCIAL PROBLEMS
- 0 1. Acts Young
- 0 11.Clings
- 0 12.Lonely*
- 1 14.Cries*
- 2 25.NotGet Along
- 1 33.Unlove*
- 2 34.OutTo Get*
- 0 35.Worth-less*
- 0 36.GetHurt*
- 2 38.Teased
- 0 48.Notliked
- 0 62.Clumsy
- 0 64.Prefers Young
- 10 TOTAL
- 68 T SCORE
- 57 CLIN T

THOUGHT PROBLEMS
- 0 9. Mind Off
- 0 18.Harms Self*
- 0 29.Fears*
- 0 40.Hears Things
- 0 66.Repeats Acts
- 0 70.Sees Things
- 0 84.Strange Behav
- 0 85.Strange Ideas
- 0 TOTAL
- 50 T SCORE
- 42 CLIN T

ATTENTION PROBLEMS
- 0 1. Acts Young
- 1 2. Hums*
- 1 4. Finish*
- 2 8.Concentr
- 2 10.SitStil
- 0 13.Confuse
- 1 15.Fidget*
- 0 17.DaDream
- 2 22.Direct*
- 2 41.Impulsv
- 1 45.Nervous
- 1 49.Learng*
- 0 60.Apath*
- 1 61 Poor School
- 0 62.Clumsy
- 2 72.Messy*
- 2 78.Inatten*
- 0 80.Stares
- 1 92.UnderAch*
- 1 100.Tasks*
- 21 TOTAL
- 61 T SCORE
- 50 CLIN T

DELINQUENT BEHAVIOR
- 2 26.NoGuilt
- 2 39.Bad Compan
- 2 43.LieCheat
- 1 63.Prefers Older
- 0 82.Steals
- 1 90.Swears
- 1 98.Tardy*
- 0 101.Truant
- 0 105.Alcohol Drugs
- 9 TOTAL
- 69 T SCORE
- 60 CLIN T

AGGRESSIVE BEHAVIOR
- 2 3. Argues
- 2 6. Defiant*
- 2 7. Brags
- 2 16.Mean
- 0 19.DemAttn
- 0 20.DestOwn
- 0 21.DestOthr
- 2 23.DisbSchl
- 2 24.Disturbs*
- 2 27.Jealous
- 2 37.Fights
- 2 53.TalksOut*
- 2 57.Attacks
- 2 67.Disrupts*
- 0 68.Screams
- 2 74.ShowOff
- 2 76.Explosive*
- 2 77.Demanding*
- 1 86.Stubborn
- 2 87.MoodChng
- 2 93.TalkMuch
- 2 94.Teases
- 2 95.Temper
- 2 97.Threaten
- 2 104.Loud
- 43 TOTAL
- 90 T SCORE
- 69 CLIN T

OTHER PROBS
- 0 5. ActOppSex
- 0 28.EatNonFood
- 0 30.FearSchool
- 0 44.BiteNail
- 0 46.Twitch
- 0 55.Overweight
- 0 56h.OtherPhys
- 0 58.PickSkin
- 0 59.SleepClass
- 2 73.Irresponsb
- 0 79.SpeechProb
- 0 83.StoresUp
- 0 91.TalkSuicid
- 0 96.SexPreocc
- 0 99.TooNeat
- 0 107.DislkSchl
- 0 109.Whining
- 0 110.Unclean
- 0 113.OtherProb

*Items not on Cross-Informant Construct

Profile Type:	WTHDR	SOMAT	SOCIAL	DEL-AGG	Att
ICC:	-.564	-.288	.242	.735**	-.180

** Significant ICC with profile type

Figure 2.1. (Continued)

29

TABLE 2.3 Cross-informant printout comparing item scores from CBCL ratings by Kyle's parents, TRF ratings by two teachers, and YSR ratings by Kyle (Actual printouts display all 89 items that have counterparts on CBCL/4-18, TRF, and YSR.)

	Mo CBC	Fa CBC	Tch TRF	Tch TRF	Slf SLF		Mo CBC	Fa CBC	Tch TRF	Tch TRF	Slf YSR
Item	1	2	3	4	5	Item	1	2	3	4	5
I WITHDRAWN						IV SOCIAL PROBLEMS					
42. Rather Be Alone	2	1	1	0	2	1. Acts Young	0	0	0	1	0
65. Won't Talk	1	2	0	0	0	11. Clings	0	2	0	0	0
69. Secretive	1	0	0	0	2	25. Not Get Along	1	1	2	1	1
75. Shy	0	0	0	0	0	38. Teased	2	1	2	1	1
102. Underactive	0	0	0	0	2	48. Not Liked	2	1	2	1	0
103. Sad	1	1	1	0	0	62. Clumsy	0	0	0	0	0
111. Withdrawn 0	0	0	0	0	2	64. Prefers Young 0	1	0	0	0	

Side-by-side comparisons of Kyle's *T* scores on the eight syndromes, Internalizing, Externalizing, and total problems are illustrated in Figure 2.3. (*T* scores are used for these comparisons because a particular *T* score indicates approximately the same degree of deviance in relation to normative samples on all scales, even though the distributions of raw scores differ from one scale to another.) As Figure 2.3 shows, the Aggressive Behavior syndrome yielded scores in the clinical range (*T* scores > 70) on ratings by both parents and both teachers. However, Kyle himself did not report more aggressive behavior than was reported by most boys in the YSR normative sample. Several items of the Aggressive Behavior syndrome that were scored 2 by multiple adult raters were scored as either 0 or 1 by Kyle. This suggests that Kyle is either less aware of these problems or is less willing to acknowledge them than are his parents and his teachers. On the other hand, Kyle's self-ratings yielded a borderline clinical *T* score of 68 on the Withdrawn syndrome. This was considerably higher than the *T* score for the Withdrawn syndrome obtained from ratings by Kyle's stepfather and teachers, although a *T* score of 65 was also obtained from his mother's ratings.

Table 2.4 shows that Kyle's scores were in the normal range on the Somatic Complaints and Attention Problems syndromes according to all five informants but that his scores were in the borderline or clinical range on the Delinquent Behavior syndrome according to three informants, on the Social Problems and Thought Problems syndromes according to two informants, and on the Anxious/Depressed syndrome according to one informant.

TABLE 2.4   Cross-informant printout comparing *T* scores from CBCL ratings by Kyle's parents, TRF ratings by two teachers, and YSR ratings by Kyle.

Scale	Mo.CBCL.1	Fa.CBCL.2	Tch.TRF.3	Tch.TRF.4	Slf.YSR.5
1. Withdrawn	65	62	57	50	68+
2. Somatic Complaints	50	53	50	50	50
3. Anxious/Depressed	63	62	69+	61	50
4. Social Problems	66	68+	68+	64	57
5. Thought Problems	76++	70+	50	65	55
6. Attention Problems	63	59	61	60	50
7. Delinquent Behavior	68+	70+	69+	59	62
8. Aggressive Behavior	79++	83++	90++	79++	61
Internalizing	62+	61+	64++	56	53
Externalizing	75++	77++	81++	71++	61+
Total Problems	71++	70++	72++	66++	55

+Borderline clinical range.
++Clinical range.

As shown at the bottom of Table 2.4, all four adult informants reported enough problems to place Kyle's total problem score in the clinical range (*T* scores > 63), but Kyle's YSR total score was well within the normal range. Coupled with Kyle's lower *T* scores on most YSR syndrome scales than on their CBCL and TRF counterparts, the overall picture indicates that interventions will need to cope with Kyle's failure to acknowledge problems that are reported by several important adults in his life.

The high levels of Externalizing problems reported by all the adult informants certainly need to be targeted for intervention. However, elevated scores on the Withdrawn, Anxious/Depressed, Social Problems, and Thought Problems scales in ratings by some informants also indicate potential complications that need to be considered in designing interventions. An initial question to be asked is whether the variations among the scores obtained from different informants indicate greater disagreements in rating Kyle than are typically found. To answer this question, the user should look at the correlations between scores obtained from the people who rated Kyle. These correlations are printed by the cross-informant program, as described in the following section.

Cross-Informant Correlations

To indicate the overall level of agreement between particular pairs of informants, the cross-informant program prints correlations between the

TABLE 2.5 Cross-informant printout of Q correlations between item scores from CBCL ratings by Kyle's parents, TRF ratings by two teachers, and YSR ratings by Kyle

For This Subject		For Reference Samples			Agreement Between:
		25th %tile	Mean	75th %ile	
Mo.CBCL.1 × Fa.CBCL.2 =	.63	.37	.51	.63	Mother and father is above average
Mo.CBCL.1 × Tch.TRF.3 =	.71	.07	.19	.30	Mother and teacher is above average
Mo.CBCL.1 × Tch.TRF.4 =	.66	.07	.19	.30	Mother and teacher is above average
Mo.CBCL.1 × Slf.YSR.5 =	.40	.22	.33	.43	Mother and youth is average
Fa.CBCL.2 × Tch.TRF.3 =	.70	.07	.19	.30	Father and teacher is above average
Fa.CBCL.2 × Tch.TRF.4 =	.56	.07	.19	.30	Father and teacher is above average
Fa.CBCL.2 × Slf.YSR.5 =	.37	.22	.33	.43	Father and youth is average
Tch.TRF.3 × Tch.TRF.4 =	.79		There is no reference sample for this combination		
Tch.TRF.3 × Slf.YSR.5 =	.36	.08	.17	.26	Teacher and youth is above average
Tch.TRF.4 × Slf.YSR.5 =	.29	.08	.17	.26	Teacher and youth is above average

item scores obtained from each pair of informants. (The correlations are known as Q correlations, which reflect the degree of similarity between sets of scores obtained from two raters. The correlations can range from −1.00, indicating perfect disagreement, to +1.00, indicating perfect agreement.) To aid users in judging how the obtained levels of agreement compare with what is typically found between informants, the program prints the 25th percentile, mean, and 75th percentile correlations found in large reference samples for similar pairs of informants. Correlations below the 25th percentile of the reference sample are designated as below average; from the 25th to 75th percentile as average; and at or above the 75th percentile as above average. Table 2.5 illustrates the cross-informant Q correlations between item scores obtained for Kyle.

By looking at the left-hand column of numbers in Table 2.5, you can see that the Q correlation between the CBCL problem items scored by Kyle's mother and stepfather was .63. By looking to the right in the same row of numbers, you can see that the correlation at the 25th percentile of the reference sample of parents was .37; the mean correlation was .51; and the 75th percentile correlation was .63. Because the correlation of .63 between the CBCL items scored by Kyle's parents was at the 75th percentile of the reference sample of parents, the printout indicates that agreement between Kyle's parents is considered above average for ratings by pairs of parents.

By looking at the correlations between each other pair of informants in Table 2.5 (i.e., the correlations below the Mo.CBCL.1 × Fa.CBCL.2 line), you can see that agreement was either average or above average for every combination of informants for which there is a reference sample. (No reference sample is provided for pairs of teachers, but the correlation of

.79 between Kyle's teachers indicates good agreement.) In addition to the correlations between item scores illustrated in Figure 2.4, the cross-informant program also prints out correlations between the syndrome scores obtained from each pair of informants, plus the 25th percentile, mean, and 75th percentile for correlations between syndrome scales in the reference samples.

SYNDROMES SCORED
FROM OTHER INSTRUMENTS

In addition to the CBCL/4-18, TRF, and YSR, syndromes have also been derived from the other empirically based instruments that are presented in this book. These instruments include the Semistructured Clinical Interview for Children and Adolescents, the Direct Observation Form, and the Child Behavior Checklist for Ages 2-3, as described in the following sections.

Semistructured Clinical Interview
for Children and Adolescents

Clinical interviews are widely used to assess children's behavioral and emotional problems (Hughes & Baker, 1990). Interviews provide unique opportunities for practitioners to interact with children, and the impressions thus gained are especially powerful. Interviews can also be used to assess children's own views of their problems and competencies, as well as to judge their interaction styles, coping strategies, and perceptions of other people. In the interview situation, the practitioner can directly observe subtle aspects of behavior that may be hard to assess by other means. A well-conducted interview can also establish a therapeutic alliance and help the practitioner judge a child's potential for responding to particular kinds of interventions. Formats for child interviews have ranged from unstructured play interviews (Irwin, 1983) to semistructured and highly structured interviews (reviewed by Hodges, 1993).

Within our multiaxial model, interviews offer one of several approaches to direct assessment of the child. Because the interview is typically limited to one context and interaction partner, the data it yields are not necessarily superior to data obtained from other sources. Instead, interview data are most useful when they can be systematically compared to data from other sources, such as parents, teachers, tests, physical examinations, and observations in other settings. Comparisons of interview data with other data can reveal variations in a child's functioning as seen by the interviewer versus other informants.

To integrate interviews with other assessment procedures, we have developed the Semistructured Clinical Interview for Children and Adolescents (SCICA; McConaughy & Achenbach, 1994b). Designed for ages 6 to 18, the SCICA provides a protocol of topics, questions, and tasks covering the nine areas outlined in Table 2.6. Unlike structured diagnostic interviews that pose yes-or-no questions about *DSM*-defined symptoms, the SCICA encourages children to express themselves freely in words and behavior. The sequence can be altered if necessary to follow the child's lead in conversation. As the SCICA proceeds, the interviewer makes brief notes on the protocol as a basis for scoring observations and the child's self-reports following the interview. Interviewers can also use audio- and videotape recordings as aids to scoring.

After the SCICA is completed, the interviewer scores the child on rating forms modeled on the CBCL and TRF. Separate sets of items are provided for scoring behavior observed during the interview and for scoring problems that the child reports during the interview. Each item is scored on the following 4-point scale: 0 if there was no occurrence; 1 if there was a very slight or ambiguous occurrence; 2 if there was a definite occurrence with mild to moderate intensity and less than 3 minutes duration; 3 if there was a definite occurrence with severe intensity or 3 or more minutes duration.

Scales for Scoring the SCICA. The SCICA provides a profile of scales for ages 6 to 12, which can be scored by hand or computer. (Research is under way to develop SCICA scales for ages 13 to 18.) To develop the SCICA scales for ages 6 to 12, interviewers and videotape observers rated 168 clinically referred children on the SCICA observation and self-report items. Principal components analyses of item scores averaged from the two raters yielded three syndromes based on children's self-reports (Aggressive Behavior, Anxious/Depressed, and Family Problems), plus five syndromes based on observations (Anxious, Attention Problems, Resistant, Strange, and Withdrawn). An Internalizing scale includes the items of the Anxious/Depressed and Anxious syndromes, whereas an Externalizing scale includes the items of the Aggressive Behavior, Attention Problems, Strange, and Resistant syndromes. The SCICA profile displays raw scores and T scores for each of the eight syndromes, plus scores for Internalizing, Externalizing, total observed problems, and total self-reported problems. The T scores compare a child's scores to those obtained by 237 clinically referred 6- to 12-year-old children. In addition,

TABLE 2.6   Topic Areas of the SCICA

I. Activities, school, job
   Favorite activities, sports, organizations
   Attitudes toward school subjects and teachers
   Homework and study strategies
   School problems
   Job (ages 13 to 18)

II. Friends
   Persons liked and disliked
   Problems with peer relations
   Social coping strategies

III. Family relations
   People in the family
   Rules, rewards, and punishments at home
   Relations with parents and siblings
   Kinetic family drawing

IV. Fantasies
   Three wishes
   Future goals

V. Self-Perceptions and Feelings
   Feelings (happy, sad, mad, scared)
   Worries
   Strange experiences

VI. Parent/teacher-reported problems
   Selected problems reported by parents on the CBCL and/or teachers on the TRF

VII. Achievement tests
   Mathematics test
   Reading recognition test

VIII. For ages 6 to 12: Screen for fine and gross motor abnormalities (optional)

IX. For ages 13 to 18: Somatic complaints, alcohol, drugs, trouble with the law

---

the SCICA manual provides mean raw scores and *T* scores for a sample of nonreferred 6- to 12-year-old children (for details, see McConaughy & Achenbach, 1994b).

SCICA for Kyle. As part of her direct assessment of Kyle, the HMO psychologist administered the SCICA. When the interview began, Kyle was withdrawn and avoided eye contact. However, as the interview progressed, he became more talkative and eager to discuss his view of his competencies and problems. As he did so, his demeanor fluctuated dramatically from cheerful and pleasant when discussing his interests and skills in sports, to intense anger when discussing conflicts with teachers and classmates. Kyle frequently complained of being treated unfairly. He felt that he was singled out for punishment in school, especially when classmates deliberately got him into trouble. He vividly recounted fights with peers, boasting that he was the strongest kid in the school. He studied karate to hone his "combat" skills. In one fight, he gave his opponent a black eye and a bloody nose. Kyle sometimes initiated fights to avenge insults or injustices, envisioning himself as the protector of weaker kids who could not fight for themselves. Other fights were sparked by "enemies" who hit him first or called him names. Because Kyle believed that his victims deserved what they got, he felt no remorse for hurting them. Kyle acknowledged breaking school rules, for example, by swearing and being in restricted areas without permission, but he said that these rules violated his rights. His school behavior often resulted in detentions, which Kyle felt were unfair.

Kyle's strategies for coping with his problems were limited mainly to physical aggression toward peers and defiance toward authority figures. Kyle did express concern about his bad temper, saying that anger swells up inside him until he loses control. However, he could not pinpoint the causes of his angry outbursts, except to say that he was either provoked by peers or treated unfairly by his teachers or parents. In addition to anger, Kyle reported sadness and worries, which mostly centered around his biological parents' divorce. Although they had divorced when he was quite young, Kyle still wished they were together. He worried about his schoolwork and his own future life. Kyle acknowledged some conflicts at home, but he felt that his mother and stepfather were much fairer than his teachers. He was especially enthusiastic about a point system at home for earning special privileges. During brief achievement tests at the end of the SCICA, Kyle complained that the math problems were hard. To keep Kyle on task, the interviewer had to repeat questions several times. Although Kyle boasted about his intellectual ability, he said he usually failed to complete homework assignments because he had too much to do. He wished he could have help with his school work like other classmates in special programs.

As shown in Figure 2.2 (on pp. 38-39), Kyle's SCICA profile had peaks on the Anxious/Depressed, Aggressive Behavior, and Strange syndromes, with scores exceeding the 90th percentile for referred children. His scores on the remaining five syndromes were closer to the 50th percentile. Kyle's scores for total observed problems and Internalizing were similar to the mean scores obtained by the SCICA clinical sample. In contrast, Kyle's scores for total self-reported problems and Externalizing were more than a standard deviation above the mean for the clinical sample. Because the SCICA scores provide comparisons with other clinically referred children, they indicated that Kyle had exceptionally severe problems in several areas.

Case Formulation for Kyle. The SCICA revealed specific aspects of Kyle's thinking that were also reflected in the elevated Thought Problems scale scores obtained from CBCLs completed by his mother and stepfather. In particular, Kyle was obsessionally preoccupied with issues of fairness and justice. Reporting considerably more aggressive behavior in the SCICA than he had acknowledged on the YSR, he justified his aggression as a struggle against the unfairness of others toward himself and toward those he protected. Thus, in addition to corroborating the aggression reported by his parents and teachers, Kyle's SCICA yielded evidence of thought distortions, extreme self-righteousness, and avoidance of responsibility for his aggression. Dramatic fluctuations in demeanor from cheerful and pleasant to intense anger graphically corroborated endorsements of the item, *Sudden changes in mood and feelings,* by both parents on the CBCL and both teachers on the TRF.

Although Conduct Disorder was the only *DSM* diagnosis for which Kyle met criteria, the empirically based procedures revealed a combination of affective volatility and paranoid ideation that would need to be considered in designing interventions. On the other hand, after some initial resistance, Kyle achieved good rapport with the SCICA interviewer, expressed great concern about his bad temper, and expressed favorable attitudes toward his mother and stepfather and their use of a point system at home. Kyle's talents in sports, interests in several hobbies, and his willingness to do chores to earn money were additional assets. At the same time, both the SCICA and an interview with Kyle's mother indicated parental inconsistency in disciplinary practices and in applying the point system. The aggressive behavior, affective volatility, and paranoid ideation argued for intensive and multifaceted interventions to ensure close coordination of behavioral management at home and school and cognitive behavioral therapy to improve his reality testing.

Direct Observation Form

In certain cases, direct observations of children in group settings are essential for comprehensive assessment. For example, evaluations of children to determine eligibility for special educational services often

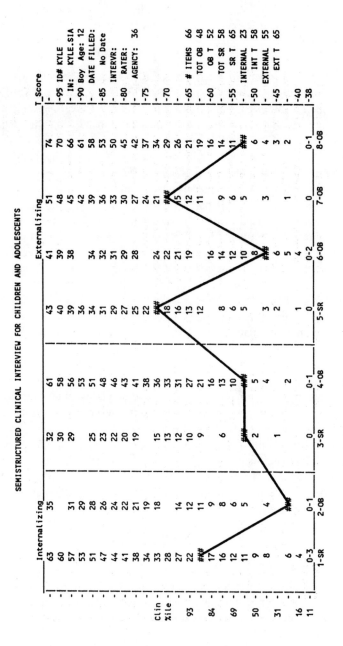

Figure 2.2. SCICA profile for 12-year-old Kyle.

ANXIOUS/DEPRESSED

- 0 128.Confused
- 0 134.Lonely
- 0 137.SelfConsc
- 0 141.Fearful
- 1 144.Concentr
- 0 146.Underact
- 2 147.Sad
- 1 157.Directns
- 0 158.Learning
- 0 160.FrMistake
- 0 162.Fears
- 0 164.Guilty
- 0 168.OutToGet
- 3 169.Overtired
- 2 171.Worthless
- 3 174.Teased
- 2 179.Nightmare
- 2 185.NotLiked
- 3 192.NGetAlong
- 0 193.NoFriends
- 2 194.SchoolWork
- 2 214.Worries
- 21 TOTAL
- 64 CLIN T

ANXIOUS

- 0 23.Confused
- 0 29.Difficlt Directns
- 0 44.Difficlt Express
- 1 46.Doesnt Remember
- 0 50.Fears Mistakes
- 0 52.Confidnc
- 0 65.Nervous
- 0 68.AnxPleas
- 0 83.SelfCons
- 0 102.TooNeat
- 0 103.Fearful
- 1 104.Tremors
- 2 TOTAL
- 44 CLIN T

FAMILY PROBLEMS

- 0 135.HarmdPar
- 0 136.Punished
- 0 142.Unfair Home
- 3 143.Unfair School
- 0 151.TooNeat
- 0 177.HatesPar
- 0 181.NoAttent
- 0 186.NotGet AlongPar
- 0 196.Screams
- 0 229.Headache
- 0 234.Stomache
- 3 TOTAL
- 54 CLIN T

WITHDRAWN

- 0 5.Apathetic
- 1 9.AvoidsEye
- 1 56.NoConver
- 0 57.NoFantsy
- 1 63.NeedCoax
- 0 72.WontTalk
- 0 73.WTFeeling
- 0 74.WontGues
- 0 77.DontKnow
- 2 79.Secretiv
- 0 80.Overtird
- 1 82.NoHumor
- 3 85.Shy
- 0 86.SlowVerb
- 0 87.SlowWarm
- 0 89.Stares
- 1 93.Stubborn
- 0 106.Underact
- 2 107.Sad
- 0 111.Quiet
- 0 114.Withdrawn
- 8 TOTAL
- 53 CLIN T

AGGRESSIVE BEHAVIOR

- 3 122.Mean
- 0 130.DisobHom
- 2 131.DisobSch
- 0 132.Impulsiv
- 0 140.suspics
- 1 145.SitStill
- 0 155.Destroys OwnThngs
- 0 156.Destroys Others
- 3 173.Fights
- 1 175.BadComp
- 3 178.HateTchr
- 1 182.NoGuilt
- 3 188.Attacks
- 3 205.Temper
- 1 207.Threaten
- 21 TOTAL
- 74 CLIN T

ATTENTION PROBLEMS

- 0 4.ActYoung
- 0 22.Concrete
- 1 24.Reverses
- 0 31.Doesnt Concentr
- 0 32.Doesnt SitStill
- 1 33.Distract
- 0 38.Fidgets
- 2 42.Clumsy
- 0 45.Understnd
- 0 53.Lapses
- 0 64.NdRepeat
- 0 66.Twitches
- 1 67.OutOfSeat
- 0 88.SpeechPrb
- 6 TOTAL
- 46 CLIN T

STRANGE

- 3 1.OverConfid
- 0 3.Giggles
- 3 15.Brags
- 1 16.BurpFart
- 2 17.MindOff
- 0 18.ChewsClth
- 0 26.Daydreams
- 0 30.Disjoint Conversat
- 3 35.Exaggerat
- 2 41.LongRespns
- 1 51.Jokes
- 0 55.Leave Toilet
- 1 71.PlaySexPrt
- 0 75.RepeatActs
- 1 91.Strange Behavior
- 1 92.MoodChange Ideas
- 1 98.Swears
- 2 100.TalkMuch
- 18 TOTAL
- 70 CLIN T

RESISTANT

- 1 6.Argues
- 0 7.AskFeedback
- 0 10.Irresponsible
- 0 14.BlameInterv
- 0 21.ComplainHard
- 1 27.Defiant
- 0 28.DemandsMet
- 0 36.Explosive
- 1 40.OffTask
- 0 43.Guesses
- 2 48.Impatient
- 1 49.Impulsive
- 0 59.OddNoises
- 0 60.MessyWork
- 1 61.Misbehaves
- 1 76.Resistant
- 0 78.Screams
- 0 84.ShowsOff
- 1 95.MoodChange
- 0 97.Suspicious
- 0 99.TalksSelf
- 1 101.TemperAngry
- 0 105.Manipulates
- 0 110.Loud
- 1 112.Quits
- 0 115.Careless
- 10 TOTAL
- 54 CLIN T

Figure 2.2. (Continued)

39

require that the children be observed in their classrooms. In other cases, marked discrepancies between reports by different teachers or between parents and teachers argue for direct observations to determine whether the child's behavior varies as much as indicated by the discrepant reports. Direct observations are also important for documenting the specific content of behavior that may not be revealed either in interviews or in reports by informants such as parents, teachers, or the children themselves. For example, the specific pattern of a child's problematic social interactions or the specific nature of hyperactive or strange behavior may be captured better by observing the child in everyday contexts than by other assessment procedures, even if the other procedures do indicate significant deviance in these areas. Furthermore, direct observations in group settings can identify behavior by others, such as peers and teachers, that may affect the child being assessed.

To combine the advantages of standardized empirically based assessment with the advantages of observing specific behaviors in everyday contexts, we have developed the Direct Observation Form (DOF; Achenbach, 1991b), which is used as follows:

1. In the space provided on the DOF, an observer writes a narrative description of the child's behavior over a 10-minute period. The description includes the behavior of others, such as peers and teachers, that impinges on the child.

2. At the end of each minute during the 10 minutes, the observer checks a box to indicate whether the child is on task at that point.

3. At the end of the 10 minutes, the on-task boxes are summed to yield a score of 0 to 10 for on-task behavior. The observer also scores 96 problem items on 4-step scales analogous to those of the SCICA. (Eighty-five of the DOF items have counterparts on the TRF, whereas 72 have counterparts on the CBC/4-18. However, all the DOF items are scored on the basis of 10-minute observational sessions, in contrast to the periods of months on which TRF and CBCL/4-18 ratings are based.)

4. The scores for the problem items are entered on the DOF profile, which includes cutpoints based on comparisons of normative and clinical samples, as described below.

5. Because children's behavior is apt to vary from one occasion to another, we recommend that 10-minute observational samples be obtained in a particular setting on three to six occasions, such as the mornings and afternoons of different days. (The computer program for scoring the DOF profile can print mean item and scale scores averaged over as many as six sessions.)

6. To provide a basis for judging the child's deviance from peers in the specific setting where the child was observed, we recommend that two "control" children of the same gender as the target child be observed, one for 10 minutes just before the target child and the other for 10 minutes just after the target child. To keep these observations relatively independent of the target child, the two control children should be located as far from the target child as possible within the same setting, such as children whose seats are on opposite sides of the room from the target child. (The DOF computer program can average the control children's scores and print them on the DOF profile for comparison with the target child's scores.)

Scales for Scoring the DOF. Analyses of DOFs for 212 clinically referred children yielded six syndromes, which are designated as With-drawn-Inattentive, Nervous-Obsessive, Depressed, Hyperactive, Attention Demanding, and Aggressive. The first three of these syndromes form an Internalizing grouping, whereas the last two form an Externalizing grouping. Because most nonreferred children manifest very few problems on any single scale, the normative data are not used to provide *T* scores but only to provide clinical cutpoints at the upper end of the distribution of scores obtained by the normative sample. The clinical range is defined as being above the 98th percentile on each syndrome scale and above the 94th percentile on the Internalizing and Externalizing scales. The distribution of total problem scores in the normative sample was sufficiently broad to provide a basis for percentiles and *T* scores, which are displayed on the DOF profile, with a clinical cutpoint at the 93rd percentile (*T* score = 65). To illustrate the DOF, we turn to the case of 7-year-old Lonnie, who will be discussed further in Chapter 5.

DOF for Case 2, Lonnie. The school psychologist in Lonnie Parker's school district had questioned whether the problems reported by Lonnie's teacher on the TRF were actually severe enough to justify a full evaluation for special education services. Because state regulations required special education evaluations to include classroom observations, the school psychologist had trained several teacher aides to use the DOF. The DOF narrative descriptions completed by a teacher aide on three occasions indicated that Lonnie continually wriggled in his seat. In addition, he often got out of his seat to crawl around on the floor behind his desk. He seldom focused on schoolwork for more than a minute. Instead, he fidgeted with pencils, erasers, and toys in his desk. He also doodled and drew pictures in his workbooks. He interrupted other children by whispering loudly to them, evoking reprimands from his teacher. Lonnie's teacher gave oral directions for each assignment and expected children to ask for help if they needed it. Lonnie occasionally asked for help, but if his teacher did not respond immediately, he became more restless and disruptive.

Figure 2.3 (on pp. 44-45) shows Lonnie's profile of DOF syndrome scores (solid line) and the mean of the syndrome scores (broken line) obtained by two control boys observed by the aide on the three occasions when she observed Lonnie. As can be seen from Figure 2.3, Lonnie's scores on the DOF Hyperactive scale were in the clinical range and well above the control boys' scores, which were in the normal range on all syndromes. Because Lonnie's scores on the other five syndromes were in the normal range, it was evident that his classroom problems were concentrated in the area tapped by the DOF Hyperactive scale. As evidence for impairment of Lonnie's classroom functioning, his on-task score was 50%, compared to a mean on-task score of 95% for the two control boys. (On-task, Internalizing, Externalizing, and total problem scores are displayed on the second page of the DOF profile, which is not shown in Figure 2.3.) According to the DOF, it thus seemed clear that Lonnie manifested significant problems of hyperactivity that interfered markedly with his schoolwork.

The Child Behavior Checklist for Ages 2-3

The Child Behavior Checklist for Ages 2-3 (CBCL/2-3) is designed to obtain ratings of children's behavioral and emotional problems from their parents and parent-surrogates. The overall format is similar to that of the problem items on the CBCL/4-18, and 59 of the 99 CBCL/2-3 problem items have counterparts on the CBCL/4-18. However, the remaining items are designed specifically for 2 and 3 year olds. Examples of these items are *Resists toilet training* and *Wanders away from home.* Because young children's behavior often changes so rapidly, the ratings are based on the preceding 2 months, rather than the 6 months used for rating problems on the CBCL/4-18.

Another difference from the CBCL/4-18 is that the CBCL/2-3 does not provide items for assessing competence in terms of activities, jobs, organizations, or school functioning, which would not be relevant for ages 2 and 3. However, like the CBCL/4-18, the CBCL/2-3 does have an open-ended item for describing the best things about the child, as well as open-ended items for describing illnesses, disabilities, and what concerns the respondent most about the child.

Scales for Scoring the CBCL/2-3. Scales for scoring the CBCL/2-3 were constructed according to the procedures outlined in Chapter 1. The samples for deriving the syndromes included 367 boys and 273 girls who were either referred for mental health services or special education services or who obtained high total problem scores in a national sample and in preschool, forensic, pediatric, and research samples (Achenbach, 1992b, provides details). Analyses for each gender separately and both genders combined yielded six syndromes that were retained as the basis for the scales of the CBCL/2-3 profile. These syndromes are designated as Anxious/Depressed, Withdrawn, Sleep Problems, Somatic Problems, Aggressive Behavior, and Destructive Behavior. Based on analyses of associations among the syndromes, an Internalizing grouping includes the Anxious/Depressed and Withdrawn syndromes, whereas an Externalizing grouping includes the Aggressive Behavior and Destructive Behavior syndromes. Percentiles and *T* scores for CBCL/2-3 scales are based on a general population sample of 368 children, with both genders combined, because gender differences in scale scores were small.

The computer program for scoring the CBCL/2-3 enables users to print side-by-side comparisons of item and scale scores obtained on up to five copies of the CBCL/2-3. This can include CBCLs filled out by the child's mother, father, and other relatives and caregivers who know the child well. It can also include CBCLs filled out by the same informant(s) on multiple occasions, such as before and after an intervention, in order to assess changes in perceived problems. Like the cross-informant program for comparing CBCL/4-18, TRF, and YSR scores, the CBCL/2-3 program computes Q correlations between the item scores obtained by each pair of up to five forms. It also prints the 25th percentile, mean, and 75th percentile Q correlations between mothers' and fathers' ratings in a reference sample, to provide a basis for judging whether obtained levels of agreement are below average, average, or above average. (Q correlations are not computed between the six syndrome scores on the CBCL/2-3, because correlations based on only six scores would be subject to too much random variation.)

In addition to informants who play parent-like roles with respect to 2- and 3-year-old children, other informants, such as preschool teachers and day care providers, may also be able to rate the many CBCL/2-3 items that are not restricted to the home situation. Because all the items of the Anxious/Depressed, Withdrawn, Aggressive Behavior, and Destructive Behavior syndrome scales can be judged on the basis of behavior outside the home, it may sometimes be useful to compare raw scores on these

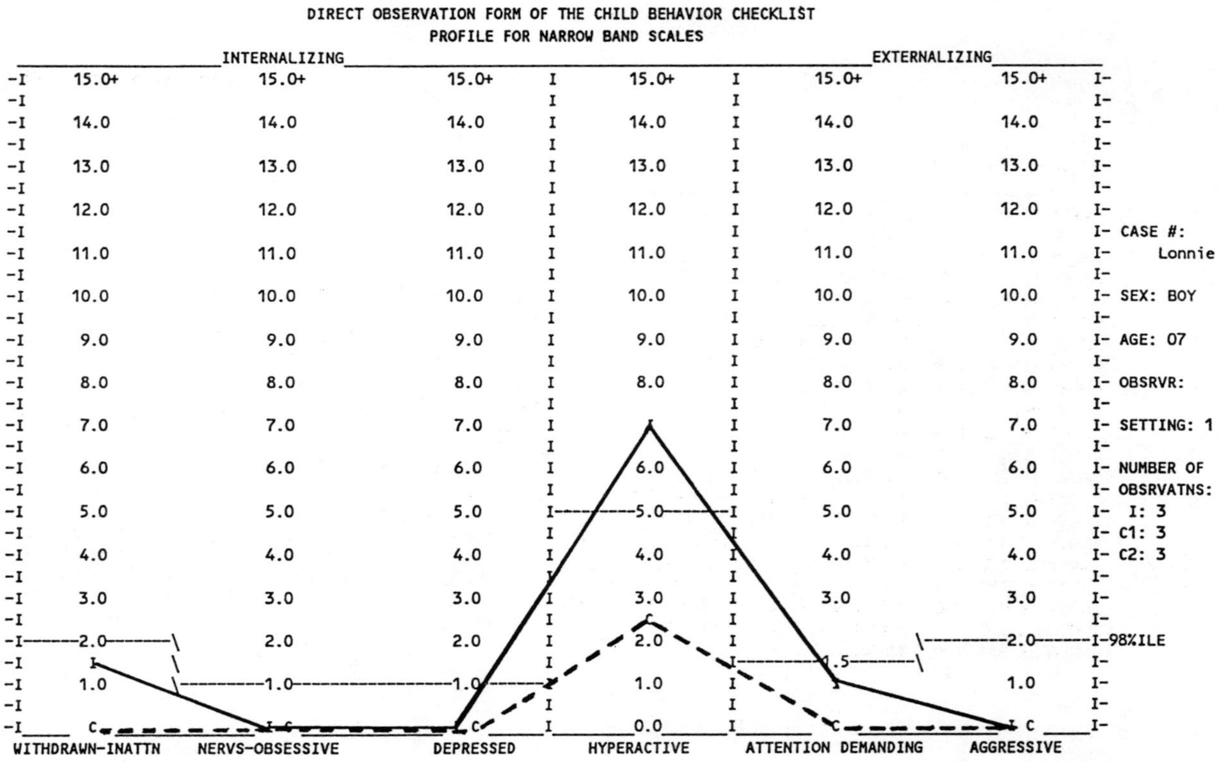

Figure 2.3. DOF profile for 7-year-old Lonnie.

I	C		I	C		I	C		I	C		I	C		I	C	
1.5	0.0	7.NO CONCNT	0.0	0.0	1.ACTS YOUNG	0.0	0.0	1.ACTS YOUNG	1.5	0.0	7.NO CONCNT	0.0	0.0	3.ARGUES	0.0	0.0	3.ARGUES
0.0	0.0	11.CONFUS	0.0	0.0	2.NOISES	0.0	0.0	28.WRTHLS	2.5	1.0	9.HYPER	0.0	0.0	5.TALK BK	0.0	0.0	5.DEFIANT
0.0	0.0	15.DAYDRM	0.0	0.0	8.OBSESS	0.0	0.0	31.TEASED	1.0	0.0	13.FIDGET	0.0	0.0	8.OBSESS	0.0	0.0	6.BRAGS
0.0	0.0	44.APATHY	0.0	0.0	11.CONFUS	0.0	0.0	37.NERVOS	0.0	0.0	33.IMPULS	0.0	0.0	10.CLINGS	0.0	0.0	14.CRUEL
0.0	0.0	57.STARES	0.0	0.0	31.TEASED	0.0	0.0	40.ANXIOS	0.0	0.0	36.NAILBT	1.0	0.0	17.WANTS ATTENTN	0.0	0.0	20.DSOBEY
0.0	0.0	75.SLOW	0.0	0.0	33.IMPULS	0.0	0.0	44.APATHY	0.5	1.0	56.DISTRA	0.0	0.0	28.WRTHLS	0.0	0.0	21.DSTURB
0.0	0.0	76.SAD	0.0	0.0	37.NERVOS	0.0	0.0	50.SLFCON	1.5	0.5	69.TALKS TOO MCH	0.0	0.0	31.TEASED	0.0	0.0	22.NO GLT
0.0	0.0	80.WITHDR	0.0	0.0	38.TWITCH	0.0	0.0	53.SHY	7.0	2.5	TOTALS	0.0	0.0	54.EXPLOD	0.0	0.0	35.LIES
			0.0	0.0	40.ANXIOS	0.0	0.0	63.STUBRN				0.0	0.0	55.FRUSTR	0.0	0.0	41.ATTACK
1.5	0.0	TOTALS	0.0	0.0	53.SHY	0.0	0.0	76.SAD				0.0	0.0	63.STUBRN	0.0	0.0	46.DISRPT
			0.0	0.0	61.STRANG BEHAV	0.0	0.0	80.WITHDR				0.0	0.0	77.LOUD	0.0	0.0	52.CLOWNS
			0.0	0.0	83.UNCLER	0.0	0.0	85.TATTLE				0.0	0.0	79.WHINES	0.0	0.0	54.EXPLOD
			0.0	0.0	91.IRRESP	0.0	0.0	89.NO GET ALONG				0.0	0.0	84.IMPATN	0.0	0.0	55.FRUSTR
						0.0	0.0	91.IRRESP				0.0	0.0	85.TATTLE	0.0	0.0	67.SWEARS
			0.0	0.0	TOTALS	0.0	0.0	95.FEARS MISTAKE				0.0	0.0	89.NO GET ALONG	0.0	0.0	70.TEASES
															0.0	0.0	73.THREAT
						0.0	0.0	TOTALS				0.0	0.0	94.COMPLN	0.0	0.0	84.IMPATN
															0.0	0.0	89.NO GET ALONG
												1.0	0.0	TOTALS	0.0	0.0	92.BOSSY
															0.0	0.0	94.COMPLN
															0.0	0.0	TOTALS

Figure 2.3. (Continued)

syndromes obtained from nonparental informants with scores obtained from parents or others who play parent-like roles with respect to a child. However, to make better use of ratings by preschool teachers and nonparental caregivers, we have developed the Teacher/Caregiver Report Form for Ages 2-5 (TCRF/2-5; Achenbach, 1995). Because of the general similarity of preschool settings for children from age 2 to 5, the TCRF/2-5 is designed to span these ages. When the construction of the scoring profile for the TCRF/2-5 is finished, it will serve as a cross-informant counterpart to the CBCL/2-3 and also to the CBCL/4-18 for assessment of children who are attending preschool, kindergarten, or day care.

INTEGRATING
CROSS-INFORMANT DATA

The multiaxial model offers a strategic framework for thinking about children's behavioral and emotional problems in terms of different facets of functioning that need to be assessed in different ways. One assessment procedure may reliably and validly capture certain aspects of a child's functioning that cannot be captured by other assessment procedures. The picture painted by each assessment procedure may reflect both situationally specific features and features that are consistent across situations. Rather than assuming that different procedures should yield the same results, we therefore need to be alert to the differences as well as the similarities between data from multiple sources. When two sources yield very different pictures of the same child, the practitioner needs to evaluate whether the differences reflect important variations in the child's functioning or differences between informants' views of functioning that is actually consistent.

In the case of Kyle, the 12-year-old boy who was presented earlier, both parents and teachers agreed in reporting high levels of aggression. However, on the Thought Problems scale, Kyle obtained a score in the clinical range on the CBCL completed by his mother and in the borderline range on the CBCL completed by his stepfather. On the TRFs completed by both teachers and the YSR completed by Kyle, the Thought Problems scale was in the normal range. The SCICA illuminated these discrepancies by revealing Kyle's extreme preoccupation with issues of fairness, his conviction that he was the strongest kid in his school, other exaggerations of his prowess, and his fantasied mission as the protector of defenseless kids. Although these features were not reported on the TRF or YSR, they were as important for understanding Kyle as were the high levels of aggression that were evident in both CBCLs, both TRFs, and the SCICA, although not in Kyle's YSR. In formulating intervention plans for Kyle, it would thus be essential to take account of features that were reported by only some informants, as well as features that were reported by most informants.

In the illustration of the DOF for 7-year-old Lonnie, the DOF provided independent documentation of the degree to which Lonnie manifested problems of hyperactivity reported by his teacher. As detailed further in Chapter 5, the combination of TRF and DOF findings supported the need for a comprehensive evaluation, which included data from Lonnie's mother, cognitive and achievement tests, and an interview with Lonnie.

Figure 2.4 presents a strategic overview of how empirically based assessment is used. The particular assessment procedures and the sequence in which they are used will vary with the setting and the specifics of the case, as illustrated in later chapters. However, the key elements of the strategy typically include:

1. gathering data from multiple sources,
2. constructing a comprehensive case formulation that takes account of similarities and differences in data, and
3. carrying out case management, including interventions, monitoring effects, and evaluating outcomes.

SUMMARY

In this chapter, we outlined strategies for using empirically based assessment data from multiple sources. Although standardized data from each source may be reliable and valid, the correlations between different sources are typically modest. Because no single source can provide the same data as all other relevant sources, comprehensive assessment requires data from multiple sources. To provide a strategic framework, a multiaxial model was presented that comprises parent reports, teacher reports, cognitive assessment, physical assessment, and direct assessment of the child, including observations in natural settings, interviews, and standardized self-report instruments.

To facilitate comparisons among parent, teacher, and self-reports, eight cross-informant syndromes have been derived from the CBCL/4-18, TRF, and YSR. A cross-informant computer program prints profiles and side-

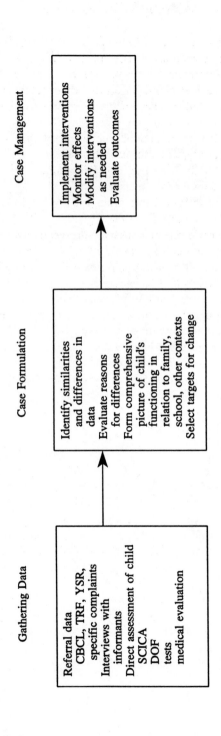

Figure 2.4. Strategic use of empirically based assessment procedures.

by-side comparisons of item and scale scores for up to five informants who have rated the same child. To provide a basis for evaluating the levels of cross-informant agreement, the program also prints Q correlations between each combination of informants for comparison with the Q correlations found in large reference samples of similar informants. To aid users in judging the degree of deviance indicated by scale scores, norms are provided for children of each gender, within particular age ranges, as rated by each type of informant. In addition to syndrome scales, scales are provided for Internalizing and Externalizing groupings of syndromes, total problems, and competencies.

The family of standardized empirically based instruments also includes the SCICA, the DOF, and the CBCL/2-3. The SCICA and DOF enable trained interviewers and observers, respectively, to sample more specific aspects of children's functioning for comparison with reports by informants who are not trained in empirically based assessment. However, owing to the limited time frames and contexts in which interviews and direct observations are feasible, the data that they yield should be judged in relation to data from other sources, rather than being considered superior to data from other sources.

The strategic use of empirically based assessment entails obtaining data from multiple sources, formulating a comprehensive picture of the case based on the multiple sources, and carrying out case management. Within this overall strategy, the particular assessment procedures and their sequence should be tailored to the setting and the specifics of the case, as illustrated in later chapters.

3

THE NATURE
AND CORRELATES OF
EMPIRICALLY BASED SYNDROMES

In Chapter 2, we introduced strategies for using empirically based assessment data from multiple informants. Cross-informant comparisons are facilitated by focusing on syndromes that have counterparts in ratings by different kinds of informants. The eight cross-informant syndromes that are scored from the CBCL/4-18, TRF, and YSR provide focal points for assessing children on the basis of data from multiple informants. The eight syndromes also provide an organizational structure for advancing research on psychopathology, as outlined in this chapter.

The empirically based syndromes represent different patterns of psychopathology in terms of the particular sets of problems that make up each syndrome. In some respects, this is analogous to the model for defining psychopathology in terms of descriptive criteria introduced by *DSM-III* and continued in *DSM-III-R* and *DSM-IV* (American Psychiatric Association, 1980, 1987, 1994). However, there are also some important differences between the *DSM* model and the empirically based syndromes.

A fundamental difference is that the *DSM* specifies fixed rules for deciding who has and who does not have each disorder. For example, the *DSM-IV* criteria for Oppositional Defiant Disorder (ODD) include a list of eight kinds of behavior, such as *Often loses temper.* To be diagnosed as having ODD, a child must be judged to manifest at least four of the eight kinds of behavior over a period of at least 6 months. In addition, the disturbance must cause clinically significant impairment in social, academic, or occupational functioning, and the behaviors must occur at times other than during a psychotic or mood disorder (pp. 93-94). A child who meets all the required criteria is judged to have ODD, whereas a child who fails to meet any of the required criteria is judged not to have ODD, regardless of the child's age or gender, or the source or completeness of the data.

The empirically based syndromes, by contrast, are designed to measure gradations in the degree to which children manifest the problems that make up a syndrome. The gradations are measured by summing the scores on the problem items of the syndrome. As a result, both the number of problems and the degree to which each problem is manifested contribute to the child's syndrome score. Normal, borderline, and clinical ranges are indicated on the scoring profiles as guides for users, but they do not imply that disorders begin and end at particular cutpoints. Nor do they require practitioners to determine the presence versus absence of disorders according to the same cutpoints for both genders, different age groups, and all sources of data. Instead, the empirically based syndromes enable users to document quantitative variations in patterns of problems.

COGNITIVE CONSIDERATIONS IN
CONCEPTUALIZING PSYCHOPATHOLOGY

In addition to the importance of quantitative gradations in judging psychopathology, there is another important reason for considering the quantitative aspects of assessment. This has to do with the ways in which human minds process information.

Some have argued that it is "natural" to think in terms of categories and that psychopathology should be diagnosed in terms of present-versus-absent categories because (a) yes-or-no decisions have to be made about care, and (b) practitioners can understand categories more easily than quantitative gradations (e.g., Angold & Costello, 1991, pp. 84-85). Yet, many decisions about care do not require just yes-or-no decisions. Instead, choices must often be made among multiple options, such as: no action; referral elsewhere; additional assessment; reassessment later; different types or combinations of treatment; short- versus medium- versus long-term interventions; and low- versus medium- versus high-intensity interventions. Furthermore, practitioners readily understand many kinds of quantitative gradations, such as scores on IQ and achievement tests, blood pressure, and body temperature.

The argument that it is more natural to think in terms of categories than gradations is also contradicted by findings that human thinking does not really conform to the traditional concept of categories (Hampton, 1993).

According to the traditional concept of categories, all members of a category are supposed to share the criterial features that define the category. Yet, even for familiar categories such as furniture, the objects that people categorize together do not all share a single set of features (Rosch & Mervis, 1975). For example, tables and chairs may share features that are not shared by other objects most people categorize as furniture, such as lamps and rugs. Furthermore, some objects may be hard to classify because they are on the border between two categories with which they share features. For example, tomatoes are hard to classify because they have features of both fruits and vegetables.

The Prototype Model

Based on a variety of findings, an alternative model has been proposed for understanding how people think about categories. Instead of portraying categorization as one-to-one matching between each defining feature of a category and the features of individual cases, the alternative model portrays categorization as a more quantitative or probabilistic process of judging the degree of similarity between the features that define a category and the features of individual cases. According to this model, a person's mental representation of a category consists of a set of imperfectly correlated features, known as a *prototype* (Hampton, 1993; Rosch, 1978).

When people judge whether a particular case corresponds to a particular prototype, they do so by assessing the degree of overlap between the features of the case and the prototypic features that define a category. Cases that have similar degrees of resemblance to two prototypes may be properly viewed as mixtures of the two prototypes or as being on the border between them. Furthermore, two cases that belong to the same category may manifest different subsets of prototypic features, rather than sharing identical sets of features with each other and with the prototypic definition of the category.

Several studies have shown that practitioners' diagnostic thinking about psychopathology actually corresponds more closely to the prototype model than to the traditional present-versus-absent model of categories (Cantor, Smith, French, & Mezzich, 1980; Horowitz, Post, French, Wallis, & Siegelman, 1981; Horowitz, Wright, Lowenstein, & Parad, 1981). Contrary to the assumption that practitioners naturally think of psychopathology in terms of present-versus-absent categories, these studies indicate that practitioners think of cases in terms of the degree to which they match diagnostic categories.

Some *DSM-IV* diagnostic categories for child psychopathology partially resemble the prototype model. For example, the *DSM-IV* criteria for Conduct Disorder (CD) include a list of 15 problem behaviors. To be diagnosed as having CD, a child must manifest at least 3 of the 15 problem behaviors, but any 3 of the 15 can qualify. Additional requirements are that "the disturbance in behavior causes clinically significant impairment in social, academic, or occupational functioning" and that "if the individual is age 18 years or older, criteria are not met for Antisocial Personality Disorder" (p. 91). Severity is to be specified as mild, moderate, or severe, depending on whether a child manifests more than the 3 problem behaviors required for the diagnosis and depending on the degree of harm caused to others. However, except for the requirement of at least 3 problem behaviors, there is no actual measure of the severity of CD in terms of the number, intensity, or frequency of the specific problems. The *DSM-IV* criteria are thus designed to classify children categorically as either having CD or not having CD according to a single cutpoint on the number of behaviors manifested.

Syndromes derived statistically from factor analytic methods are quite analogous to conceptual prototypes (Hampton, 1993). Like conceptual prototypes, the syndromes consist of problems that tend to occur together, although their co-occurrence is not so uniform that each problem is always accompanied by all the others.

When used for empirically based assessment, each factor-analytically derived syndrome is scored quantitatively to reflect gradations in the degree to which the problems composing a syndrome are reported for an individual. This contrasts with the *DSM* practice of imposing a single fixed cutpoint on a list of problem items. Despite this and other differences between the empirically based and *DSM* approaches to psychopathology, the prototype model should be kept in mind as a conceptual bridge between these approaches. As illustrated by findings presented in this chapter, there are numerous points of contact between the empirically based and *DSM* approaches. Furthermore, even some of the differences between the approaches can spur dialogues that may ultimately advance our understanding of psychopathology.

COMORBIDITY ISSUES

Comorbidity refers to the coexistence of two or more disorders in the same person. When *DSM-III* introduced explicit criteria for diagnosing the presence versus absence of disorders, it was soon found that many children qualified for multiple diagnoses (Costello, Edelbrock, Dulcan, Kalas, & Klaric, 1984). This stimulated research on the rates and implications of comorbidity among childhood disorders (e.g., Caron & Rutter, 1991). The rates of comorbidity between some *DSM* diagnoses are so high as to raise questions about whether they really represent separate disorders. For example, two studies have reported 96% comorbidity between CD and ODD, whereas a third study has reported 84% comorbidity between them (Faraone, Biederman, Keenan, & Tsuang, 1991; Spitzer, Davies, & Barkley, 1990; Walker, Lahey, et al., 1991). Because the *DSM* requires decisions about whether each disorder is present versus absent, children who meet diagnostic criteria for multiple disorders are concluded to have each of the disorders.

In addition to revealing high comorbidity rates, studies of comorbidity among *DSM* disorders have been complicated by the fact that they typically compute comorbidity in only one direction. That is, they start with Disorder A and then tabulate the proportion of individuals having Disorder A who also have Disorder B. However, if the number of individuals having Disorder A differs from the number having Disorder B, the comorbidity computed from A to B will differ from the comorbidity found by starting with individuals who have Disorder B and then tabulating those who also have Disorder A.

To illustrate problems arising from this unidirectional computation of comorbidity, McConaughy and Achenbach (1994a) used a bidirectional procedure to recompute comorbidities that had been reported in four studies of *DSM* diagnoses of children. The bidirectional procedure obtains the mean of the unidirectional computation of comorbidity from Diagnosis A to B and from Diagnosis B to A. When the bidirectional procedure was applied to the four studies, it yielded quite different comorbidity rates than had been obtained by the various unidirectional computations from either Diagnosis A to B or B to A. Reports of comorbidity between *DSM* diagnoses may thus be distorted by arbitrarily categorizing children according to one diagnosis and then tabulating how many children meet criteria for another diagnosis.

Because the empirically based syndromes are scored on quantitative scales and children receive scores on all syndromes, comorbidity does not raise issues of the sort encountered with *DSM* diagnoses. Instead, a child's profile of syndrome scores provides a picture of the child's standing on all syndromes, as rated by a particular informant. The child's profiles scored from ratings by other informants provide additional pictures to be compared, contrasted, and integrated with each other. Deviant scores on multiple syndromes indicate that a child has a variety of problems. However, profile patterns that reveal a variety of problems do not force us to choose between disorders or to decide which disorders are comorbid with which other disorders. If we wish to know the degree to which a particular syndrome tends to co-occur with other syndromes, we can compute correlations between syndrome scores in particular samples of children. We can also compute the degree to which deviance on one syndrome tends to co-occur with deviance on other syndromes in terms of odds ratios between them. (Odds ratios indicate the odds of a particular outcome, such as a deviant score on Syndrome B, for individuals having a particular characteristic, such as deviance on Syndrome A, compared to individuals not having that characteristic.)

Profile Types

Children's profiles often indicate that they have mixtures of various kinds of problems. Some of these mixtures may be unique to particular children, as seen by particular informants. Other mixtures may be reflected in patterns that characterize substantial numbers of children. To identify such patterns, we have performed cluster analyses of the CBCL/4-18, TRF, and YSR profiles of large samples of children referred for mental health services. These cluster analyses identified types of profile patterns that are shared by particular subsets of children. A detailed presentation of the profile types and their correlates has been published elsewhere (Achenbach, 1993).

To indicate the degree to which a child's profile resembles each of the types identified through cluster analysis, the lower left corner of the computerized printout of the CBCL/4-18, TRF, and YSR profiles displays intraclass correlations between the child's profile and the profile types found for children of that gender and age. A correlation above .44 indicates a statistically significant degree of resemblance to a profile type. Where relevant, the case illustrations in Chapters 5 through 7 will discuss the resemblance of particular children's profiles to the profile types.

We turn now to findings related to the eight cross-informant syndromes that are central foci of our approach to empirically based assessment. For convenience, we will proceed alphabetically among the three syndromes of the Internalizing grouping, followed by the two syndromes of the

Externalizing grouping, and then the three syndromes that are not included in either of these groupings.

INTERNALIZING SYNDROMES

Beginning with research findings in the 1960s (Achenbach, 1966), the term *internalizing* was chosen to describe a broad class of co-occurring problems that mainly involve inner distress, in contrast to *externalizing* problems, which mainly involve conflicts with others and with social mores. The Internalizing grouping of cross-informant syndromes includes the Anxious/Depressed, Somatic Complaints, and Withdrawn syndromes. The correlations found among these syndromes do not mean that children who score high on one of these syndromes inevitably score high on the other two syndromes. Nor are high scores on the Internalizing syndromes inevitably accompanied by low scores on the Externalizing syndromes. Some children have both kinds of problems, as well as problems that are not classified as Internalizing versus Externalizing.

For purposes of clinical management, it is often useful to know whether a child's problems are primarily internalizing or externalizing. Nevertheless, although the Internalizing syndromes have certain features in common that differ from features common to the Externalizing syndromes, there are also important differences among the three syndromes of the Internalizing grouping and between the two syndromes of the Externalizing grouping. Thus, scores on specific syndromes are often more informative than the global distinction between internalizing and externalizing.

The Anxious/Depressed Syndrome

As was shown in Table 2.2, the Anxious/Depressed syndrome that was found in CBCL/4-18, TRF, and YSR ratings includes items that are indicative of anxiety, such as *Too fearful or anxious*. This syndrome also includes items indicative of depressed affect, such as *Unhappy, sad, or depressed*. Other items of the syndrome may be associated with both anxiety and depression, such as *Cries a lot*. By contrast, the *DSM* assigns anxiety disorders and depressive disorders to separate categories. It is also customary to distinguish between anxiety versus depressive responses to particular events. For example, an event that threatens harm is expected to evoke anxiety, whereas an event involving loss, such as the death of a loved one, is expected to evoke depression. However, among people who display such emotions chronically in the absence of specific traumatic events, it may be harder to draw a clear boundary between anxiety and depression.

It may be especially hard to draw a clear boundary between chronic anxiety and depression in children. This difficulty is illustrated by the fact that measures of anxiety and depression both use similar items (King, Ollendick, & Gullone, 1991). For example, the item, "I often worry about something bad happening to me," serves as a measure of anxiety on the Revised Children's Manifest Anxiety Scale (RCMAS; Reynolds & Richmond, 1978). Yet, the very similar item, "I worry that bad things will happen to me," is included in the Children's Depression Inventory (CDI; Kovacs, 1981). Even when more distinctive measures of anxiety and depression are used, problems intended to measure anxiety versus depression tend to co-occur and to have similar biological correlates (Finch, Lipovsky, & Casat, 1989).

In addition to ambiguities about which problems reflect anxiety versus depression, developmental sequences further complicate the relations between them. For example, longitudinal findings indicate that childhood problems that initially meet criteria for anxiety disorders are later followed by problems that meet criteria for depressive disorders (Kovacs, Gatsonis, Paulauskas, & Richards, 1989). It is also possible that some assessment procedures are more sensitive to the overlap between anxiety and depression, whereas other procedures are more sensitive to the differences between them. For example, children's self-reports on the SCICA have yielded a syndrome designated as Anxious/Depressed, which includes a combination of anxiety and depressive items resembling the cross-informant Anxious/Depressed syndrome (McConaughy & Achenbach, 1994b). By contrast, interviewers' observational ratings have yielded a syndrome designated as Anxious, because it is composed exclusively of SCICA items that are indicative of anxiety. Another syndrome derived from interviewers' observational ratings includes SCICA items that are indicative of depressed demeanor, although this syndrome is designated as Withdrawn, because items indicative of withdrawal had the highest loadings in the factor-analytic derivation of the syndrome.

The degree of separation between signs of depression and anxiety may thus depend on the source of data, with children's self-reports blending both kinds of affect to a greater extent than interviewers' observations. It is possible that the observational differences between the SCICA syndromes designated as Anxious and Withdrawn primarily reflect children's reactions to the interview context, whereas parent, teacher, and self-reports reflect more persistent patterns that are evident outside the interview context.

Negative Affectivity. Even in adults, it has been hard to draw clear boundaries between persistent anxiety and depressive problems. Genetic studies of adults have shown that Generalized Anxiety Disorder and Major Depression are influenced by the same genetic factors (Kendler, Neale, Kessler, Heath, & Eaves, 1992; Kendler et al., 1995). This suggests that vulnerabilities to anxiety and depression are closely related, even though environmental factors may shape the ways in which they are manifested.

To elucidate the strong associations between anxiety and depression, it has been proposed that both are manifestations of *negative affectivity* (Watson & Clark, 1984). This refers to a general disposition to experience discomfort across diverse situations that are not stressful for most people. The difficulty of distinguishing between persistent anxiety and depression may therefore arise partly from the fact that they both reflect a general disposition to negative affect. This view is not intended to account for all problems of anxiety or depression. In fact, among children who score high on the cross-informant Anxious/Depressed syndrome, some may have high scores primarily on the anxiety items, some primarily on the depressive items, some on the items that are hard to classify (such as *Cries a lot*), and some on other combinations of the items. Furthermore, Watson, Clark, and their coworkers have provided evidence that adult self-report measures can distinguish negative affectivity both from physiological hyperarousal symptoms that are thought to indicate anxiety and from anhedonia, which is thought to indicate depression (Watson, Clark, et al., 1995; Watson, Weber, et al., 1995).

Coherence of the Anxious/Depressed Syndrome. Despite possible differences among subsets of anxiety and depressive items, the cross-informant Anxious/Depressed syndrome shows high internal consistency, as indicated by Cronbach's alpha coefficients ranging from .86 to .90 across all the gender/age groups on the CBCL/4-18, TRF, and YSR (Achenbach, 1991b, 1991c, 1991d). These high internal consistencies indicate that the relations among the subsets of anxiety, depressed, and mixed items are quite strong within the cross-informant Anxious/Depressed syndrome. Furthermore, longitudinal analyses of a representative national sample showed 3-year correlations averaging .46 across parent, teacher, and self-ratings of the Anxious/Depressed syndrome among children and adolescents (Achenbach, Howell, McConaughy, &

Stanger, 1995a). Over a 3-year period of transition from adolescence to young adulthood, the longitudinal correlations averaged .57 for parent and self-ratings (Achenbach, Howell, McConaughy, & Stanger, 1995c). Moreover, regression analyses indicated that early scores on the Anxious/ Depressed syndrome greatly outweighed other syndromes, competencies, family variables, and intervening events (e.g., stressful experiences) as 3-year predictors of later scores on the Anxious/Depressed syndrome among both adolescents and young adults. Further research may clarify the extent to which anxiety and depressive disorders should be separated, but the Anxious/Depressed syndrome has been well-supported as a coherent pattern of problems over the age range from which it was derived.

Relations to Other Assessment Procedures. Several studies have analyzed relations between the empirically based Anxious/Depressed syndrome and various diagnostic criteria. For example, Rey and Morris-Yates (1992) used Receiver Operating Characteristic (ROC) analyses to test the relation of syndrome scores to *DSM* diagnoses that were made from the clinical case histories of disturbed Australian adolescents. They found that Anxious/Depressed syndrome scores from both the CBCL/4-18 and YSR discriminated well between adolescents who met *DSM* criteria for Major Depression versus other disorders.

In addition to *DSM* diagnoses made from case histories, *DSM* diagnoses based on other data have been significantly associated with the empirically based Anxious/Depressed syndrome. For example, in a Puerto Rican community sample, Gould, Bird, and Jaramillo (1993) analyzed the relations of diagnoses made from a combination of parent and child psychiatric interviews to Anxious/Depressed syndrome scores obtained by averaging CBCL/4-18 and YSR standard scores. Significant associations were found between the Anxious/Depressed syndrome scores and *DSM-III* diagnoses of Overanxious and Separation Anxiety disorders. Furthermore, a study of adolescent inpatients found significant associations between the pre-1991 version of the YSR Depressed syndrome and *DSM* diagnoses of both affective and anxiety disorders made from psychiatric interviews (Weinstein, Noam, Grimes, Stone, & Schwab-Stone, 1990). (The pre-1991 YSR Depressed syndrome correlates .89 to .96 with the 1991 YSR Anxious/Depressed syndrome; Achenbach, 1991c)

Significant correlations have also been found between the empirically based syndrome and measures that are not structured according to *DSM* criteria. For example, parents' CBCL ratings on the pre-1991 Depressed syndrome (which correlates .96 to .99 with the 1991 CBCL Anxious/

Depressed syndrome; Achenbach, 1991b) were found to correlate .51 with depression scores obtained by children in a semistructured clinical interview, the Child Assessment Schedule (CAS; Hodges, Kline, Stern, Cytryn, & McKnew, 1982). In addition, scores on the Behavior Assessment System for Children (BASC) parent and teacher scales for Anxiety and Depression have correlated from .52 to .84 with the CBCL and TRF Anxious/Depressed scales (Reynolds & Kamphaus, 1992).

Relations to Maternal Depression. Associations have been found between mothers' CBCL ratings of their children's problems and measures of the mothers' own depression (e.g., Conrad & Hammen, 1989; Friedlander, Weiss, & Traylor, 1986; Richters & Pellegrini, 1989). These associations have led some to suggest that depression may distort mothers' judgments of their children's problems. However, in a comprehensive review of relevant research, Richters (1992) concluded that "None of the studies that claimed evidence for a depression→distortion influence on mothers' ratings of their children met the necessary and sufficient criteria for establishing distortion" (p. 485). Instead, studies that used other informants to provide external checks on mothers' ratings showed that depressed mothers agreed with the other informants at least as well as nondepressed mothers did.

There is considerable evidence from sources other than mothers' ratings that children of depressed mothers actually do have more problems than children whose mothers are not depressed. Children whose mothers are depressed may have elevated rates of problems for several reasons. Examples include the following: (a) children's problems and their mothers' depression could both be reactions to a common stressor, such as abuse by fathers; (b) children's problems may be responses to their mothers' depression; (c) children may share their mothers' learned and/or constitutional vulnerabilities to depression; and (d) mothers' depression may be a response to elevated problem levels in their children.

Associations between parent and child problem scores have also been found for problems other than depression, for fathers as well as for mothers, and for child problem scores on measures completed by other informants, such as the TRF completed by teachers (Brown et al., 1993; Jensen, Traylor, Xenakis, & Davis, 1988). Thus, when associations are found between informants' characteristics and their reports about children, their reports should not be automatically dismissed as distortions. Instead, such associations may contribute important information about the informants as well as about the children.

The Somatic Complaints Syndrome

The Somatic Complaints syndrome comprises physical problems without known medical causes. Examples include headaches, stomachaches, and vomiting. The Somatic Complaints syndrome resembles the *DSM* diagnostic category of Somatization Disorder, although *DSM-IV* does not list Somatization Disorder among disorders that are usually first evident in infancy, childhood, and adolescence. Lacking a specific childhood category for somatic complaints, *DSM-IV* does include such complaints among the symptoms that may be present in Separation Anxiety Disorder. That is, physical complaints in response to separation from attachment figures can count toward the symptoms required for a diagnosis of Separation Anxiety Disorder, but physical symptoms are not specifically required for the diagnosis.

Although somatic complaints may indeed occur in response to separation anxiety, our analyses have yielded a clear-cut syndrome of somatic complaints that does not include direct manifestations of anxiety. Furthermore, the CBCL/2-3 has yielded a syndrome of somatic problems that is similar to the syndrome derived from parent, teacher, and self-ratings for both genders on the CBCL/4-18, TRF, and YSR. In addition, a fairly similar syndrome has been identified in parent ratings and young adult self-ratings on the Young Adult Behavior Checklist (YABCL) and Young Adult Self-Report (YASR), respectively.

Moderate developmental continuity between somatic complaints syndromes identified on the different instruments is indicated by a 3-year correlation of .41 between syndrome scores on the CBCL/2-3 at age 3 and on the CBCL/4-18 at age 6 (Achenbach, 1992b). Across the transition from adolescence to adulthood, a similar level of developmental continuity is evident in a mean correlation of .43 obtained by averaging longitudinal correlations from the CBCL/4-18 to the YABCL versions of the syndrome and from the YSR to the YASR versions across a 3-year period (Achenbach et al., 1995c). Furthermore, studies of twins have yielded heritabilities of .50 and .63 for the CBCL/2-3 Somatic Problems syndrome and .51 and .73 for the CBCL/4-18 Somatic Complaints syndrome (Edelbrock, Rende, Plomin, & Thompson, 1995; Schmitz, Fulker, & Mrazek, 1995; van den Oord, Verhulst, & Boomsma, 1996). There is thus considerable evidence for a pattern of somatic complaints that is manifest from early childhood to young adulthood, that has moderate developmental continuity, and that is significantly influenced by genetic factors.

Relations to Other Assessment Procedures. Perhaps because of the lack of a childhood equivalent of Somatization Disorder in the *DSM,* few studies have focused on syndromal patterns of somatic complaints among children. In one of the few studies, Routh and Ernst (1984) compared 7 to 17 year olds who had abdominal pain from physical illness to a group who had abdominal pain without detectible physical causes. The group whose pain had no detectible physical causes obtained significantly higher scores on the pre-1991 CBCL Somatic Complaints syndrome than did the group whose pain did have known physical causes. (The pre-1991 CBCL Somatic Complaints syndrome correlates .90 to .95 with the 1991 CBCL syndrome; Achenbach, 1991b.) The difference between the groups was specific to the CBCL Somatic Complaints syndrome, as the groups did not differ significantly on any other CBCL problem scale.

Additional findings in the Routh and Ernst (1984) study suggested a familial genetic vulnerability to somatization that is consistent with the substantial heritabilities cited earlier. In particular, among the 20 children whose abdominal pain resulted from a known physical cause, only 1 (5%) had a close relative who met *DSM* criteria for Somatization Disorder. This was significantly less than the 50% rate found for children whose abdominal pain had no known physical cause.

In other research, a correlation of .42 was obtained between parents' ratings on the pre-1991 CBCL Somatic Complaints syndrome and self-ratings by 8 to 17 year olds on the Children's Somatization Inventory (CSI; Walker, Garber, & Greene, 1991). The CSI, which is designed to assess somatic symptoms that are not attributable to physical causes, comprises 36 symptoms that are read to the child and are then rated by the child on four-step scales. Parents' ratings on the 1991 CBCL Somatic Complaints syndrome have also correlated .70 with parents' ratings on the Psychosomatic Scale of the Conners (1973) Parent Questionnaire (Achenbach, 1991b).

In a study where measures of pain were partialled out, children with migraine headaches scored significantly higher on the CBCL Somatic Complaints syndrome than did children suffering pain from musculoskeletal abnormalities and a no-pain control group (Cunningham et al., 1987). The Somatic Complaints syndrome thus appears to reflect a general tendency to report somatic problems independent of the level of pain that may actually be experienced.

The Withdrawn Syndrome

The problem items of the Withdrawn syndrome mainly reflect disengagement from other people, low energy, and some negative affectivity. *DSM-III* and *DSM-III-R* both included a diagnostic category for Avoidant Disorder of Childhood or Adolescence that implied a pattern resembling the Withdrawn syndrome but that did not provide specific descriptive features. However, *DSM-IV* does not include this diagnostic category. Instead, it provides a category for Avoidant Personality Disorder, which is intended primarily for adults.

Despite the omission of Avoidant Disorder of Childhood or Adolescence from *DSM-IV,* there is a substantial body of research on shyness and withdrawal as aspects of temperament that may predict later behavioral and emotional problems (e.g., Kagan, 1994). Furthermore, counterparts of the Withdrawn syndrome have been found in analyses of the CBCL/2-3, the YABCL, and the YASR (Achenbach, 1992b; Achenbach et al., 1995c). Developmental continuity between the successive versions of the Withdrawn syndrome is indicated by a 3-year correlation of .46 for the CBCL/2-3 version at age 3 with the CBCL/4-18 version at age 6, and a mean 3-year correlation of .53 for adolescent CBCL/4-18 and YSR versions with adult YABCL and YASR versions. Furthermore, scores on the Withdrawn syndrome discriminate strongly between children referred for mental health services and nonreferred peers (Achenbach, 1991b, 1991c, 1991d, 1992b).

Relations to Other Assessment Procedures. The pre-1991 version of the CBCL Withdrawn syndrome was found to be significantly associated with *DSM-III* diagnoses of Avoidant Disorder of Childhood or Adolescence, Major Depression, Dysthymia, and Separation Anxiety (Edelbrock & Costello, 1988; Gould et al., 1993). (The pre-1991 CBCL version of the Withdrawn syndrome correlates .90 to .98 with the 1991 CBCL/4-18 version; Achenbach, 1991b.) In addition, the 1991 cross-informant syndrome scored from a combination of parent and self-ratings has been found to correlate significantly with *DSM-III* diagnoses of Dysthymia and Separation Anxiety made from a combination of parent and child psychiatric interviews in the Puerto Rican community sample studied by Gould et al. (1993). There are thus significant points of contact between the Withdrawn syndrome and several *DSM* diagnostic categories, but no single *DSM-IV* category captures the overall pattern of problems composing the Withdrawn syndrome.

A moderate degree of genetic influence on the Withdrawn syndrome has been indicated by a heritability estimate of .50 among the 7- to 15-year-old twins studied by Edelbrock et al. (1995) and .40 among the 4- to 11-year-old twins studied by Schmitz et al. (1995). The genetic factors may operate through hormonal mechanisms, as CBCL/4-18 and YSR scores on the Withdrawn syndrome have been found to predict cortisol levels following psychologically challenging interactions better than did numerous other variables for clinically referred children (Granger, Weisz, & Kauneckis, 1994).

EXTERNALIZING SYNDROMES

Separate second-order factor analyses of the eight cross-informant syndromes for each gender in each age range of the CBCL/4-18, TRF, and YSR yielded a factor on which the Aggressive Behavior and Delinquent Behavior syndromes had the highest loadings. The problems that make up these Externalizing syndromes are often referred to collectively as conduct problems. In fact, the *DSM-IV* diagnostic category of CD includes a mixture of behaviors like those of the Aggressive Behavior syndrome, such as fighting and cruelty, with behaviors like those of the Delinquent Behavior syndrome, such as lying, stealing, truancy, and running away from home. In addition, *DSM-IV* assigns some problems like those of the Aggressive Behavior syndrome to the separate category of ODD. Examples include *Loses temper* and *Argues*.

Although many of the items of the Aggressive Behavior and Delinquent Behavior syndromes have counterparts among the descriptive features of the *DSM* categories of CD and ODD, the *DSM* categories do not reflect the distinction between overt aggression and more covert violations of social mores that has long been identified in many studies beside our own (e.g., Hewitt & Jenkins, 1946; Jenkins & Boyer, 1968; Loeber & Schmaling, 1985; Quay, 1986). In fact, because a *DSM-IV* diagnosis of CD requires the presence of only 3 out of 15 descriptive features, some children who qualify for the diagnosis manifest exclusively aggressive behavior, whereas others manifest exclusively nonaggressive delinquent behavior, and still others manifest both kinds of behavior. *DSM-IV* diagnoses of CD may therefore mask important differences between the types of conduct problems that children manifest.

The Aggressive Behavior Syndrome

Patterns of co-occurring problems like those of the Aggressive Behavior syndrome have been found in many samples of children, assessed by different procedures, and analyzed in different ways. In addition, aggressive behavior problems show substantial continuity between developmental periods. A 3-year longitudinal correlation of .54 has been obtained between the CBCL/2-3 Aggressive Behavior syndrome at age 3 and the CBCL/4-18 version of this syndrome at age 6 (Achenbach, 1992b). Over the transition from adolescence to young adulthood, a mean 3-year longitudinal correlation of .55 has been obtained from the CBCL/4-18 to the YABCL and from the YSR to the YASR versions of the syndrome (Achenbach et al., 1995c). Although not involving our empirically based Aggressive Behavior syndrome, significant correlations have been found between peer nominations for aggression at age 8 and several measures of aggression at age 30 (Eron & Huesmann, 1990). Teachers' ratings of aggression at age 10 have also been found to predict criminal offenses up to age 26 in a Swedish longitudinal study (Stattin & Magnusson, 1989).

Genetic studies of the CBCL/4-18 Aggressive Behavior syndrome have yielded heritability estimates of .94 among 4- to 7-year-old twins (Ghodsian-Carpey & Baker, 1987), .55 among 4- to 11-year-old twins (Schmitz et al., 1995), and .60 among 7- to 15-year-old twins (Edelbrock et al., 1995). A heritability estimate of .70 was obtained in a different type of study of CBCL Aggressive Behavior syndrome scores in 10- to 15-year-old children from several countries who had been adopted by Dutch parents (van den Oord, Boomsma, & Verhulst, 1994). Furthermore, longitudinal genetic analyses indicated that 100% of the genetic influences are the same for the Aggressive Behavior syndrome scored on the CBCL/2-3 for preschoolers and on the CBCL/4-18 for the same children at 4 to 11 years old (Schmitz et al., 1995). The Schmitz et al. study obtained a heritability estimate of .52 for the Aggressive Behavior syndrome scored from the CBCL/2-3, whereas a version of the Aggressive Behavior syndrome scored from the CBCL/2-3 for Dutch twins yielded a heritability of .69 (van den Oord et al., 1996).

The genetic findings suggest important biological influences on the Aggressive Behavior syndrome. One model for representing such biological influences has been proposed by Quay (1993) on the basis of Gray's (1982, 1987a, 1987b) theory of the Behavioral Inhibition System (BIS) and the Reward System (REW) of brain function. Quay has hypothesized that people with aggressive conduct disorders have a relatively inactive

BIS. Furthermore, Quay cites behavioral studies indicating that people with aggressive conduct disorders persevere excessively in trying to win payoffs despite very high odds against success, such as with lottery jackpots. According to Quay, these findings suggest a dominance of the REW system, as well as a weak BIS, in people who are persistently aggressive. Quay's model is one way of thinking about possible biological factors in the Aggressive Behavior syndrome, but other models may also be useful for understanding the growing body of evidence for biological factors, as summarized in the following sections.

Relations to Other Assessment Procedures. As indicated earlier, *DSM-III-R* and *DSM-IV* do not distinguish aggressive from nonaggressive CD. However, *DSM-III* distinguished among subcategories designated as Undersocialized Aggressive, Undersocialized Nonaggressive, Socialized Aggressive, and Socialized Nonaggressive CD. In a clinical sample, Edelbrock and Costello (1988) found that scores on the CBCL Aggressive Behavior syndrome were more strongly associated with *DSM-III* diagnoses of Aggressive CD than Nonaggressive CD. In a community sample of Puerto Rican children, Gould et al. (1993) obtained too few diagnoses of CD for separate analyses of the *DSM-III* Aggressive versus Nonaggressive subtypes of CD. However, they found a significant relation between diagnoses of ODD and Aggressive Behavior syndrome scores, where both the diagnoses and syndrome scores were based on combinations of parent and self-reports. Thus, when reports of aggressive behavior are rare, as in the Gould et al. community sample, diagnoses of ODD may reflect relatively mild levels of the problems that are included in the Aggressive Behavior syndrome better than do diagnoses of CD, at least according to *DSM-III* criteria.

In addition to associations with *DSM* diagnoses, the Aggressive Behavior syndrome has been found to correlate highly with scales from other rating instruments. For example, Conduct Problem scores from the Conners (1973) and Quay-Peterson (Quay & Peterson, 1982) parent rating instruments have correlated .86 and .88, respectively, with CBCL/4-18 Aggressive Behavior syndrome scores (Achenbach, 1991b). Similarly, Conduct Problem scores from the Conners Revised Teacher Rating scale (Goyette, Conners, & Ulrich, 1978) have correlated .80 with TRF Aggressive Behavior syndrome scores (Achenbach, 1991b). Scores on the BASC parent and teacher Aggression scales have correlated .58 to .89 with the CBCL/4-18 and TRF Aggressive Behavior scores (Reynolds & Kamphaus, 1992).

Consistent with the genetic evidence for biological factors in the Aggressive Behavior syndrome, several studies have found significant associations between biochemical measures and syndrome scores. Three studies have reported significant negative correlations of –.50, –.63, and –.72 between measures of serotonergic activity and CBCL Aggressive Behavior syndrome scores in children (Birmaher et al., 1990; Hanna, Yuwiler, & Coates, 1995; Stoff, Pollock, Vitiello, Behar, & Bridger, 1987). These findings are consistent with the theory that low serotonergic activity is quantitatively related to high aggression (Brown & van Praag, 1991).

A correlation of –.81 has been found between dopamine-beta-hydroxylase (DBH) levels and CBCL Aggressive Behavior syndrome scores (Gabel, Stadler, Bjorn, Shindledecker, & Bowden, 1993). In addition, a correlation of .47 has been found between Aggressive Behavior scores on the TRF and testosterone levels measured in saliva (Scerbo & Kolko, 1994). Although much more needs to be known about the relations between various biochemical parameters and aggressive behavior, scores on the Aggressive Behavior syndrome are clearly associated with biological differences among children.

The associations between Aggressive Behavior scores and biological factors do not necessarily mean that environmental factors play no role nor that levels of aggressive behavior cannot be reduced. On the one hand, environmental factors such as stress may cause biochemical reactions that affect aggressive behavior, although the biochemical reactions themselves are apt to be affected by genetic factors. On the other hand, a clear understanding of relations between environmental, biochemical, and genetic factors may provide a better basis for treatment of aggression than we have to date.

Distinguishing Between Aggressive and Nonaggressive Conduct Problems

Unfortunately, there has been a tendency to lump overtly aggressive and covertly delinquent behavior together as conduct problems, antisocial behavior, or juvenile delinquency. Insensitivity to differences between kinds of conduct problems may impede our understanding of environmental and intervention effects that might differ for the Aggressive Behavior versus Delinquent Behavior syndromes. The syndromes may also follow different developmental courses.

As an example, in addition to the Aggressive Behavior and Delinquent Behavior syndromes, our analyses of the YABCL and YASR have identified a young adult syndrome designated as Shows Off (Achenbach et al., 1995c). The Shows Off syndrome is composed mostly of the socially intrusive but not physically aggressive items of the pre-adult Aggressive Behavior syndrome. These items include: *Showing off* (the item that loads highest on the Shows Off syndrome), *Bragging, Demands attention, Talks too much, Teases a lot,* and *Unusually loud.* Scores on the pre-adult Aggressive Behavior syndrome have been the best predictors of scores on the young adult Shows Off syndrome in both a national sample and a clinical sample (Achenbach et al., 1995c; Stanger, MacDonald, McConaughy, & Achenbach, 1996). This indicates that some aggressive youths become less physically aggressive in early adulthood while still retaining their socially intrusive behavior. It also suggests that, despite the evidence for traitlike stability and genetic factors in the Aggressive Behavior syndrome, other factors may tip the balance away from the most aggressive aspects of the syndrome. In any event, it is important to avoid lumping aggressive and intrusive behavior with the kind of covert violations of social mores represented by the Delinquent Behavior syndrome, to which we now turn.

The Delinquent Behavior Syndrome

As was shown in Table 2.2, the problems of the Delinquent Behavior syndrome involve violations of social mores that are not characterized by aggressive and intrusive behaviors like those of the Aggressive Behavior syndrome. Aggressive and delinquent behaviors do co-occur often enough to cause the two syndromes to obtain similar mean loadings of .79 and .78, respectively, on the second-order factor designated as Externalizing. However, children may be deviant on one syndrome without being deviant on the other syndrome. For example, averaged across parent, teacher, and self-ratings, only 28% of children in a national sample who were deviant on one of the syndromes were also deviant on the other syndrome. Even in a clinical sample, the corresponding figure was only 45% (McConaughy & Achenbach, 1994a).

There are also developmental differences between the aggressive and delinquent syndromes. Although similar versions of the Aggressive Behavior syndrome have been found from age 2 through adulthood, some behaviors of the Delinquent Behavior syndrome are simply not relevant to preschool ages, such as truancy and use of alcohol or drugs. The irrelevance of such behaviors may account for the failure to find a counterpart of the Delinquent Behavior syndrome in the CBCL/2-3 (Achenbach, 1992b). On the other hand, some behaviors of the delinquent syndrome also become less relevant at older ages. Examples include truancy after the age when compulsory education ends and use of alcohol after the age when it becomes legal. Nevertheless, the YABCL and YASR have yielded a Delinquent Behavior syndrome among young adults. This syndrome includes adult counterparts of the truancy and alcohol use items, such as *Stays away from school or work when not sick or not on vacation* and *Drinks too much alcohol or gets drunk.* Thus, a pattern of violations of social mores is also evident in adulthood, even though societal standards for defining violations differ from those that apply to younger ages. Furthermore, a mean 3-year correlation of .49 has been obtained from the CBCL/4-18 and YSR to the YABCL and YASR versions of the Delinquent Behavior syndrome (Achenbach et al., 1995c).

In addition to lacking a counterpart prior to age 4, the Delinquent Behavior syndrome has shown relatively low longitudinal correlations of .40, .40, and .36 over 2, 4, and 6 years, respectively, in a general population sample of Dutch children (Verhulst & van der Ende, 1992). These correlations were all significantly lower than the correlations of .67, .63, and .55 found for the Aggressive Behavior syndrome over the same periods in the same sample. The less traitlike nature of the delinquent than the aggressive syndrome is also suggested by the heritability estimates of .35 (not statistically significant) obtained by Edelbrock et al. (1995) and .39 obtained by van den Oord et al. (1994) for the Delinquent syndrome versus .60 and .70 for the Aggressive syndrome in the same studies. An exception to these findings was a heritability of .79 obtained for Delinquent Behavior in a study of 4- to 11-year-old twins, where the heritability of Aggressive Behavior was .55 (Schmitz et al., 1995).

Relations to Other Assessment Procedures. The tendency to lump delinquent behaviors with aggressive behaviors as conduct problems in diagnoses and other assessment procedures makes it difficult to test their relations to the Delinquent Behavior syndrome, which does not include overtly aggressive behavior. However, in a study of relations between the YSR and diagnoses made from Diagnostic Interview Schedule for Children (DISC) interviews with adolescent inpatients, YSR Delinquent Behavior syndrome scores had a considerably stronger association than Aggressive Behavior syndrome scores with *DSM-III* diagnoses of CD, most of which were of the nonaggressive subtype (Weinstein et al., 1990).

In the Puerto Rican community sample studied by Gould et al. (1993), the Delinquent Behavior syndrome scored from combined CBCL/4-18 and YSR data was more strongly associated than the Aggressive Behavior syndrome with *DSM-III* diagnoses of CD made from combined parent and child interview data. On the BASC parent and teacher rating forms, which have separate scales for aggression and conduct problems, the BASC conduct problems scale has correlated from .76 to .93 with CBCL/4-18 and TRF Delinquent Behavior syndrome scores (Reynolds & Kamphaus, 1992). The Delinquent Behavior syndrome has also been found to be a strong predictor of police contacts in a national sample, especially for girls (Achenbach, Howell, McConaughy, & Stanger, 1995b).

Although they did not necessarily operationalize delinquent behavior in the same way as does the cross-informant Delinquent Behavior syndrome, studies reviewed by Quay (1993) indicate that—unlike aggressive youths—youths with delinquent behavior problems do not differ from other youths in moral reasoning, abstract reasoning, empathy, stimulus seeking, or psychophysiological responses. Unaggressive delinquent youths have also been found to adapt better to institutional settings and to have better outcomes after release from these settings than do aggressive youths (Henn, Bardwell, & Jenkins, 1980).

Another aspect of the differences between the Delinquent Behavior and Aggressive Behavior syndromes is that they appear to follow different developmental trajectories. In CBCL ratings of Dutch children assessed five times at 2-year intervals, scores on both syndromes declined from ages 4 to 10 (Stanger, Achenbach, & Verhulst, 1996). However, after about age 10, scores on the Delinquent Behavior syndrome increased until about age 17, whereas scores on the Aggressive Behavior syndrome declined. Furthermore, significantly more children changed from being nondeviant to being deviant on the delinquent than the aggressive syndrome. These changes from nondeviant to deviant scores on the Delinquent Behavior syndrome occurred significantly more often among adolescents than among younger children.

Coupled with the significantly higher longitudinal correlations found for the Aggressive than the Delinquent syndrome (e.g., Verhulst & van der Ende, 1992), the above findings suggest differences like those hypothesized by Moffitt (1993) between life-course persistent and adolescence-limited antisocial behavior. According to Moffitt's hypothesis, a combination of biological and environmental risk factors leads to antisocial behavior that some people persistently manifest throughout childhood and into adulthood. A contrasting developmental pattern occurs among relatively normal youths who temporarily manifest increases in antisocial behavior during adolescence. These temporary increases are more apt to reflect adolescent developmental issues and peer influences than long-term psychopathology. Although further research is needed to obtain a more precise picture, the evidence to date suggests that the Aggressive Behavior syndrome is more characteristic of the life-course persistent developmental pattern, whereas the Delinquent Behavior syndrome is more characteristic of the adolescence-limited pattern. Consistent with this view, a New Zealand general population sample showed an adolescent increase in *DSM-III* diagnoses of nonaggressive conduct disorders but not aggressive conduct disorders (McGee, Feehan, Williams, & Anderson, 1992).

SYNDROMES NOT CLASSIFIED AS INTERNALIZING OR EXTERNALIZING

The Attention Problems, Social Problems, and Thought Problems syndromes were not associated exclusively enough with either of the second-order Internalizing and Externalizing factors to warrant including them in either of these groupings. This does not mean that the Attention Problems, Social Problems, and Thought Problems syndromes form a separate grouping analogous to the Internalizing and Externalizing groupings. Instead, deviant scores on these syndromes are apt to occur either alone or in combination with deviant scores on any of the cross-informant syndromes. Because our second-order factor analyses did not reveal a separate grouping of these three syndromes, we do not aggregate their scores into a global score as we do with those for the Internalizing and Externalizing groupings.

The Attention Problems Syndrome

As was shown in Table 2.2, the Attention Problems syndrome includes problems of inattention, overactivity, and impulsivity. Besides the 10 items that define the cross-informant construct, the TRF Attention Problems scale includes 10 additional items that teachers are especially likely to observe and that loaded on the TRF version of the Attention Problems syndrome. Examples of the items specific to the TRF Attention Problems scale include the following: *Hums or makes other odd noises in class, Fails to finish things he/she starts, Fidgets,* and *Difficulty following directions.*

Attention Problems syndrome scores have shown substantial developmental continuity. For example, CBCL/4-18 scores have yielded longitudinal correlations of .60 over 2 years, .56 over 4 years, and .44 over 6 years in a Dutch general population sample (Verhulst & van der Ende, 1992). In our American national sample, a mean longitudinal correlation of .54 was obtained for CBCL/4-18, TRF, and YSR ratings over a 3-year period (Achenbach et al., 1995a).

Although the longitudinal correlations for the Attention Problems syndrome are substantial between the ages of 4 and 18, our analyses of the CBCL/2-3 did not yield a clear counterpart of this syndrome in younger children (Achenbach, 1992b). Our failure to find an Attention Problems syndrome for ages 2 and 3 was not apt to result from a lack of appropriate items on the CBCL/2-3. Six of the 10 items of the cross-informant Attention Problems syndrome appear on the CBCL/2-3, plus the following items that could potentially be associated with such a syndrome in young children: *Can't stand waiting, wants everything now; Demands must be met immediately;* and *Quickly shifts from one activity to another.* The closest approximation to the Attention Problems syndrome in the CBCL/2-3 is a syndrome designated as Destructive Behavior, which includes *Can't concentrate, can't pay attention for long,* and *Quickly shifts from one activity to another.* However, the other nine items of this syndrome are not clear analogues of items that make up the Attention Problems syndrome. Factor analysis of Dutch children's scores on the CBCL/2-3 has yielded a small syndrome designated as Overactive, but it differs considerably from the Attention Problems syndrome found for older children (Koot, 1993). Because prolonged attention is not expected of very young children, attention problems may not form a clear-cut syndrome at ages 2 and 3.

The possibility of attention disorders in adulthood has received a great deal of publicity (e.g., Cowley & Ramo, 1993), but no official diagnostic criteria have been published for adult versions of these disorders. In our analyses of parents' YABCL ratings of their young adult offspring, we have identified a syndrome that includes counterparts of six items from the Attention Problems syndrome construct. Designated as Irresponsible, this young adult syndrome includes additional items such as *Irresponsible behavior* (the highest loading item), *Has trouble making decisions, Fired from a job,* and *Feels he/she can't succeed.* The syndrome does not include items indicative of hyperactivity, but research on children diagnosed as having *DSM-III-R* Attention Deficit Hyperactivity Disorder (ADHD) indicates that hyperactivity declines in adolescence, whereas attention problems do not decline (Hart, Lahey, Loeber, Applegate, & Frick, 1995). A mean longitudinal correlation of .62 over a 3-year period from CBCL/4-18 Attention Problems scores to YABCL Irresponsible scores in young adulthood indicates considerable developmental continuity between these two syndromes (Achenbach et al., 1995c). Tests of multiple candidate predictors also showed that adolescent Attention Problems scores were the strongest predictors of YABCL Irresponsible scores. The Irresponsible syndrome thus appears to reflect a continuation into adulthood of the problems represented by the Attention Problems syndrome.

Evidence for genetic influences on the Attention Problems syndrome has been provided by heritability estimates of .56, .65, .66, .72, and .79 in twin studies (Edelbrock et al., 1995; Gjone, Stevenson, & Sundet, 1996; Schmitz et al., 1995; Zahn-Waxler, Schmitz, Fulker, Robinson, & Emde, 1996). Among 10- to 15-year-old international adoptees raised by Dutch parents, van den Oord et al. (1994) obtained a heritability estimate of .47 for the CBCL Attention Problems syndrome.

Relations to Other Assessment Procedures. The Attention Problems syndrome includes several items similar to the criterial features of the *DSM-III, DSM-III-R,* and *DSM-IV* versions of ADHD. However, these *DSM* versions of ADHD have differed considerably in structure and criteria. *DSM-III* provided three separate lists of features for inattention, impulsivity, and hyperactivity. A *DSM-III* diagnosis of ADD with Hyperactivity required features from all three lists, whereas a diagnosis of ADD without Hyperactivity required features from only the first two lists. In a major departure from *DSM-III, DSM-III-R* provided a single list of 14 features, from which 8 were required for a diagnosis of ADHD. In a further departure, *DSM-IV* provides separate lists of 9 features for inattention and 9 for hyperactivity/impulsivity. At least 6 features from each list are required for a diagnosis of ADHD, Combined Type. If 6 features are present from only the inattentive list, the diagnosis is ADHD, Predominantly Inattentive Type. On the other hand, if 6 features are present from only the hyperactivity-impulsivity list, the diagnosis is ADHD, Predominantly Hyperactive-Impulsive Type.

As a result of the major changes in diagnostic criteria, different children qualified for the *DSM-III* versus *DSM-III-R* versions of ADHD (Lahey et al., 1990). The major changes from *DSM-III-R* to *DSM-IV* are also likely to result in different children qualifying for diagnoses, with a variety of relations possible between the three *DSM-IV* ADHD subtypes and the one *DSM-III-R* ADHD type. Several studies have found significant associations between both *DSM-III* and *DSM-III-R* diagnoses and the Attention Problems syndrome scored from the CBCL/4-18, TRF, and YSR (e.g., Barkley, DuPaul, & McMurray, 1990; Edelbrock & Costello, 1988; Gould et al., 1993; Steingard, Biederman, Doyle, & Sprich-Buckminster, 1992; Weinstein et al., 1990).

ROC analyses have shown that the CBCL/4-18 Attention Problems scale achieved almost perfect accuracy in identifying children who were independently diagnosed as having ADHD at any time in their lives, according to *DSM-III-R* criteria (Chen, Faraone, Biederman, & Tsuang, 1994). The accuracy also remained extremely high when the Attention Problems cutpoint based on clinically referred children was applied to their brothers and sisters. As Chen et al. pointed out, the diagnostic accuracy of the Attention Problems scale equaled or exceeded the accuracy of widely used biomedical tests for physical illnesses.

Despite the differences in their structure, content, and derivation, the Attention Problems syndrome and the various *DSM* ADHD criteria thus identify many of the same children. It remains to be seen how strongly scores on the Attention Problems syndrome relate to the three ADHD subtypes of *DSM-IV*. In addition to their associations with *DSM-III* and *DSM-III-R* criteria, the CBCL/4-18 and TRF Attention Problems scales also show moderate to high correlations with analogous scales of the Conners parent and teacher questionnaires, the Quay-Peterson Revised Behavior Problem Checklist, and the BASC (data are presented by Achenbach, 1991b, 1991c; Reynolds & Kamphaus, 1992).

Gender Differences in Attention Problems. According to *DSM-IV* (p. 82), ADHD is much more common in males than females, with ratios ranging between 4 to 1 in general population samples and 9 to 1 in clinics. Perhaps because ADHD is assumed to be a mainly male disorder, most studies have included few, if any, females (e.g., Mannuzza, Klein, Bessler, Malloy, & LaPadula, 1993). When females have been included, their data have often been combined with the male data for analysis. As a result, most findings related to diagnoses of ADHD are based mainly on males.

Rather than applying the same diagnostic cutpoint to both genders, our empirically based approach employs syndrome scores that are analyzed and normed separately for males and females. This facilitates testing associations between attention problems and other variables across the entire range of variation actually found for each gender. The importance of considering each gender separately is highlighted by the distribution of scores found in our national normative sample. Despite the exclusion of children who were receiving mental health or special education services, scores on the TRF Attention Problems scale in our national normative sample were considerably lower for girls than boys. For example, the 98th percentile score on the TRF Attention Problems scale for ages 5 to 11 is 29 for boys, compared to 24 for girls. If a diagnostic cutpoint were chosen on the basis of the boys' scores, few girls would be identified as deviant on the Attention Problems syndrome. However, when we performed separate multiple regression analyses of the girls and boys in our national sample, we found stronger predictive relations from early to later scores on the Attention Problems syndrome for girls than boys (Achenbach et al., 1995a).

Our longitudinal analyses also showed that the Attention Problems syndrome predicted a greater variety of later syndrome scores for girls than boys, including Social Problems, Thought Problems, Delinquent Behavior, and Aggressive Behavior (Achenbach et al., 1995a). In addition, multiple regression analyses yielded stronger predictive relations between adolescent Attention Problems scores and young adult Irresponsible scores for females than males (Achenbach et al., 1995c). These findings are consistent with evidence for greater brain metabolism abnormalities found in pre-adult and adult females than males who were diagnosed as having ADHD (Ernst et al., 1994). It is not yet known whether the findings for females with attention problems reflect more impairment, a developmentally more persistent trait, or lower rates of treatment because females who have attention problems may be less likely than males to be recognized as needing help. In any event, rather than assuming that females do not have attention problems merely because they fail to meet diagnostic criteria based mainly on males, we need to compare attention problems reported for individual females with those reported for normative samples of females.

The Social Problems Syndrome

As was shown in Table 2.2, the Social Problems syndrome consists of items indicative of immaturity and a lack of social skills. This syndrome has no clear counterpart in *DSM-IV,* but empirically based analyses of various rating forms have identified counterparts in at least 13 samples of children (Achenbach, 1992a). In a collaborative study of syndromes derived from the American and Dutch CBCLs and the American Achenbach, Conners, Quay Behavior Checklist, a counterpart syndrome was identified that was designated as Socially Inept (Achenbach, Conners, Quay, Verhulst, & Howell, 1989). Correlations of .78 to .98 have been obtained between the Social Problems syndrome and pre-1991 syndromes that were designated as Unpopular on the TRF and YSR and as Social Withdrawal and Hostile Withdrawal on the CBCL (Achenbach, 1991b, 1991c, 1991d).

Moderate longitudinal stability has been found for the Social Problems syndrome, as indicated by a mean 3-year correlation of .46 averaged over CBCL, TRF, and YSR ratings, and correlations of .49, .38, and .33 in CBCL ratings by Dutch parents over 2, 4, and 6 years, respectively (Verhulst & van der Ende, 1992). Substantial genetic influence has been found in twin studies where the heritability estimates have been .56 and .61 (Edelbrock et al., 1995; Schmitz et al., 1995). In addition, a young adult version of the Social Problems syndrome was found in parents' YABCL ratings. Predictive correlations from adolescent CBCL scores to adult YABCL scores on the Social Problems syndrome averaged .45 over a 3-year period in a national sample (Achenbach et al., 1995c).

Relations to Other Assessment Procedures. Despite the lack of a specific *DSM* counterpart, the Social Problems syndrome has been significantly associated with *DSM-III* diagnoses of ADHD and Overanxious Disorder, based on data combined from parent and self-reports (Gould et al., 1993).

Exceptionally good cross-informant agreement has been found among ratings of the Social Problems syndrome by mothers, fathers, teachers, and youths. In an Australian sample of 11 to 16 year olds, the Social Problems syndrome yielded a mean correlation of .62 for self-ratings with parent and teacher ratings (Sawyer, 1990; data presented by Achenbach, 1991d). This was higher than was found for any other cross-informant syndrome. Such good agreement for self-ratings by youths with ratings by their parents and teachers is remarkable, because the Social Problems syndrome is composed of items that are apt to be hard for some youths to acknowledge, such as *Acts too young for age, Too dependent, Gets teased, Not liked,* and *Clumsy.* Mean correlations of .77 between mothers' and fathers' ratings of Social Problems and .65 between parents' and teachers' ratings also reflected exceptionally high cross-informant agreement (Achenbach, 1991b, 1991c).

For agreement in classifying children as being in the normal versus borderline and clinical ranges on the Social Problems syndrome, odds ratios between the CBCL and TRF, the CBCL and YSR, and the TRF and YSR ranged from 9.5 to 11.0, which were well above the odds ratios for any other syndromes scored from these combinations of instruments (Achenbach, 1991a). The Social Problems syndrome has also yielded relatively high odds ratios for discrimination between referred and non-referred children on the CBCL (odds ratio = 10.9) and TRF (odds ratio = 8.3; Achenbach, 1991b, 1991c).

Among children who received mental health services, deviant CBCL Social Problems scores at intake were exceptionally good predictors of deviant YSR Social Problems scores at follow-up assessments averaging 4.9 years later, as shown by an odds ratio of 9.1 (Stanger, MacDonald, et al., 1996). This further indicates exceptionally good agreement between parent and youth reports of problems that are likely to be hard for some youths to acknowledge, in this case over an interval averaging 4.9 years for youths who were deviant enough to be referred for mental health services.

The lack of counterparts for the Social Problems syndrome in the official diagnostic system and in other assessment procedures has tended to limit research on it to date. However, the exceptionally good cross-informant agreement in ratings of the Social Problems syndrome, as well as its demonstrated strength in discriminating between referred and non-referred children, argue for focusing more closely on it as an index of impairment and a target for interventions.

The Thought Problems Syndrome

Some problems of this syndrome tend to be rare among normal and mildly deviant children, especially *Hears sounds or voices that aren't there* and *Sees things that aren't there*. Other items are somewhat more common but may encompass quite diverse content, such as *Strange behavior* and *Strange ideas*. The remaining items of the Thought Problems syndrome, *Can't get mind off certain thoughts* and *Repeats certain acts over and over*, are fairly common, especially in self-reports on the YSR. Both for scoring purposes and for purposes of clinical interpretation, all the foregoing items request respondents to describe the problems that they score as present. This enables practitioners to determine whether what is reported should be counted as the respondent has scored it, should be scored on a different item that is more specific to the content, or should not be scored at all.

To help parents and teachers understand the target problems for *Can't get mind off certain thoughts,* the word *obsessions* is included with the CBCL/4-18 and TRF versions. Similarly, the word *compulsions* is included with *Repeats certain acts over and over* on the CBCL/4-18 and TRF. However, the words obsessions and compulsions are not included on the YSR, because adolescents are not expected to understand them in relation to their own thoughts and acts. Furthermore, it is helpful for practitioners to obtain adolescents' self-reports about any repetitive thoughts and acts, whether or not they meet clinical criteria for obsessions or compulsions. It is not assumed that everything scored as present on these items reflects clinically deviant obsessions or compulsions. Nor is it assumed that everything scored as present on the other items of the syndrome reflects hallucinations, delusions, or extreme deviance. Instead, the scored items may include mild versions of these problems, some of which might be evaluated as subclinical when considered alone. However, the higher the overall score on the Thought Problems syndrome, the greater the evidence that the child may have clinically deviant thought problems.

Prior to the derivation of the cross-informant Thought Problems syndrome, most of its items were on pre-1991 syndromes that were designated as Schizoid, Obsessive-Compulsive, or Thought Disorder, depending on the instrument and the gender/age group. The correlations between the 1991 Thought Problems syndrome and the pre-1991 versions range from .81 to .92 (Achenbach, 1991b, 1991c, 1991d). Syndromes resembling the Thought Problems syndrome have been found in empirically based analyses of at least 22 samples (Achenbach, 1992a). However, there has been considerable variation among the items composing these syndromes, depending on the instruments that were used, the raters, and the prevalence of the constituent problems among the children who were rated.

Heritability estimates of .44 and .56 have been obtained in twin studies (Edelbrock et al., 1995; Schmitz et al., 1995). This indicates that there is significant genetic influence on even the relatively low scores found on this scale in nonclinical samples.

Relations to Other Assessment Procedures. The Quay-Peterson Revised Behavior Problem Checklist (Quay & Peterson, 1982) is one of the few commonly used rating forms that has an empirically based scale—designated as Psychotic—that resembles the Thought Problems scale. Parents' ratings on the Quay-Peterson Psychotic scale have correlated .64 with the CBCL/4-18 Thought Problems scale (Achenbach, 1991b).

The closest *DSM* counterpart to the Thought Problems syndrome is Schizotypal Personality Disorder. The Thought Problems syndrome also includes features of Obsessive-Compulsive Disorder and some psychotic disorders. These diagnoses are rare in children, but the Gould et al. (1993) community study of Puerto Rican children found significant associations between the Thought Problems syndrome and four other *DSM* diagnoses, including ODD, Simple Phobia, Overanxious Disorder, and Dysthymia, where syndrome ratings and diagnoses were based on combined parent and child data. Although Gould et al. did not analyze Schizotypal, Obsessive-Compulsive, or psychotic disorders, their findings indicate that relatively high scores on the Thought Problems syndrome were associated with a broad array of diagnosed psychopathology.

In a comparison between girls diagnosed as having Obsessive-Compulsive Disorder and girls having trichotillomania (compulsive hair pulling), the girls with Obsessive-Compulsive Disorder scored much higher on the CBCL/4-18 Thought Problems scale (mean $T = 75$) than girls with trichotillomania (mean $T = 65$). However, the girls with trichotillomania scored significantly higher than other clinically referred girls (mean $T = 60$; King et al., 1995). Despite the fact that trichotillomania is defined by compulsive hair pulling, the Thought Problems scores obtained by these girls were nevertheless considerably lower than the Thought Problems scores obtained by girls who were diagnosed as having a more generalized Obsessive-Compulsive Disorder. In a sample that included both sexes, children who were diagnosed as having Obsessive-Compulsive Disorder obtained a mean T score of 77 on the CBCL/4-18 Thought Problems syndrome, which was very similar to the mean of 75 found by King et al. for girls with Obsessive-Compulsive Disorder (Hanna, 1995).

Using the pre-1991 CBCL/4-18 Schizoid scale, which correlates .81 to .86 with the CBCL/4-18 Thought Problems scale, Bergman and Walker (1995) found that children of schizophrenic parents had significantly higher scores than children whose parents had other psychiatric conditions and a control group whose parents were considered normal.

Because of the low prevalence rates of most items on the Thought Problems syndrome, relatively low total scores on this syndrome can reach the clinical range. This is especially true on the CBCL/4-18 and TRF, where a score of 4 falls at the 98th percentile clinical cutpoint for both genders at all ages. On the YSR, a score of 8 for boys and 9 for girls falls at the 98th percentile clinical cutpoint. Because the presence of so few problems (e.g., two items scored 2 on the CBCL/4-18 and TRF) indicates deviance, it is important to avoid overinterpreting deviant scores on the Thought Problems syndrome. Users should therefore examine the descriptions written by respondents for the items that they have scored present and should inquire about them in order to ascertain whether the scores are justified. Inquiries are also necessary to ascertain the context in which the problems occur in order to evaluate the evidence for thought problems. If it is clear that deviant scores are justified, more extensive evaluation will be needed to determine whether a psychotic or serious obsessive-compulsive disorder is present. However, there is mounting evidence that high scores on the Thought Problems syndrome do indicate serious psychopathology.

SUMMARY

Cognitive research has demonstrated that people tend to categorize individual cases by judging the degree to which features of each case correspond to sets of features that define each category. People thus conceptualize categories as sets of imperfectly correlated features, known as prototypes.

The empirically based syndromes operationally define prototypic patterns of psychopathology in terms of problems found to be mutually correlated. The degree to which a child manifests a syndrome is indicated by the syndrome score. Children can obtain high scores on a syndrome by manifesting any subset of the syndrome's items, each of which partially measures the prototypic pattern composing the syndrome. Furthermore, any pattern of high and low scores on the profile of syndrome scales can occur without requiring forced choices between disorders or raising co-morbidity issues.

Viewing the cross-informant syndromes as eight prototypic patterns of psychopathology, we presented research findings that illuminate the nature and correlates of each syndrome. The Anxious/Depressed syndrome includes some items that are primarily indicative of anxiety, some that are primarily indicative of depression, and some that may be associated with both types of affect. The combination of anxiety and depression in a single syndrome is consistent with evidence for a general disposition to experience negative affect, which may be manifested by both kinds of symptoms.

Several studies have found significant associations between the Anxious/Depressed syndrome and *DSM* diagnoses of both anxiety and depressive disorders, as well as with non-*DSM* criteria. Associations of CBCL/ 4-18 Anxious/Depressed syndrome scores with maternal depression have led some to suggest that mothers' depression distorts their judgments of their children's problems. However, evidence does not support the depression→distortion hypothesis, as depressed mothers' ratings of their children agree with ratings by other informants at least as well as ratings by nondepressed mothers.

The Somatic Complaints syndrome has shown moderate continuity across developmental periods beginning at age 3 and continuing into young adulthood. Significant genetic influences are indicated by findings from twin studies and by a strong association with elevated rates of Somatization Disorder in family members. Scores on the Somatic Complaints syndrome also correlate significantly with several measures of somatic symptoms that are not attributable to physical causes.

The Withdrawn syndrome has been significantly associated with several *DSM* diagnoses, including the *DSM-III* diagnosis of Avoidant Disorder of Childhood or Adolescence. However, *DSM-IV* retains only Avoidant Personality Disorder, which is intended primarily for adults. Moderate developmental continuity has been found for the Withdrawn syndrome over periods from age 3 to early childhood and extending into early adulthood. Twin studies indicate moderate genetic influence, which may operate through hormonal mechanisms, such as high cortisol levels.

The Aggressive Behavior syndrome shows strong continuity over developmental periods ranging from the early preschool years to adulthood. Heritability estimates ranging from .52 to .69 for the CBCL/2-3 and from .55 to .94 for the CBCL/4-18, plus significant correlations with biochemical parameters, indicate important biological factors. The Aggressive Behavior syndrome is significantly associated with diagnoses of CD and ODD, but *DSM-III-R* and *DSM-IV* dropped the *DSM-III* distinction between aggressive and nonaggressive conduct disorders. The most recent editions of the *DSM* thus lack a distinction that has been supported by many kinds of research and that is reflected in the differences between the Aggressive Behavior and Delinquent Behavior syndromes. In young adulthood, the socially intrusive behaviors of the Aggressive Behavior syndrome form a separate syndrome designated as Shows Off, which is strongly predicted by adolescent scores on the Aggressive Behavior syndrome. Some aggressive youths may thus become less physically aggressive while retaining their socially intrusive behavior.

Characterized largely by covert violations of social mores, the Delinquent Behavior syndrome shows less developmental continuity than the Aggressive Behavior syndrome, as well as less evidence for genetic or other biological correlates. Increases in conduct problems during adolescence may mainly involve the Delinquent Behavior syndrome, whereas the Aggressive Behavior syndrome has more traitlike stability across developmental periods.

Between the ages of 4 and 18, scores on the Attention Problems syndrome show strong developmental continuity. After age 18, parents' YABCL ratings have yielded a syndrome designated as Irresponsible that is significantly predicted by adolescent Attention Problems scores and that includes items indicative of difficulties in assuming adult responsibilities. Genetic influences on the Attention Problems syndrome are indicated by heritability estimates ranging from .47 to .72. Scores on the Attention Problems syndrome have been significantly associated with *DSM* diagnoses of ADHD. Gender-specific scores on the Attention Problems syndrome predict a greater variety of later problems among females than males. This argues for using gender-specific scores and cutpoints to identify attention problems, rather than criteria that are based mainly on males and that identify few females.

Comprising items indicative of immaturity and poor social skills, the Social Problems syndrome does not have a clear counterpart in *DSM-IV.* However, it has been significantly associated with *DSM-III* diagnoses of ADHD and Overanxious Disorder. Substantial genetic influence is indicated by heritability estimates of .56 and .61. Exceptionally good cross-informant agreement has been found among ratings of the Social Problems syndrome by mothers, fathers, teachers, and youths.

Most children obtain very low scores on the Thought Problems syndrome. As a result, endorsement of only a few items can produce scale scores in the clinical range, especially on the CBCL/4-18 and TRF. Because respondents are asked to describe the problems that they endorse, practitioners should look at the descriptions to ensure that the scores are appropriate and also to provide a starting point for clinical interviewing about the problems. Despite the low scores, heritability estimates of .44 and .56 indicate significant genetic influence. Research has revealed high scores on the CBCL/4-18 Thought Problems scale for children who were diagnosed as having Obsessive-Compulsive Disorder, as well as significant associations with a variety of other *DSM* diagnoses.

4

APPLYING EMPIRICALLY BASED ASSESSMENT

Chapter 3 presented the prototype model for conceptualizing patterns of psychopathology. The empirically based syndromes operationally define prototypic patterns of psychopathology whose nature and correlates differ in ways such as those outlined in Chapter 3. In preparation for illustrating applications of empirically based assessment to individual children, this chapter provides an overview of how the procedures are used in various contexts.

GATHERING DATA

When requesting evaluation of children's behavioral and emotional problems, parents and teachers often state their concerns in global terms such as hyperactivity, learning problems, or "doesn't get along with others." When asked for details, they may recount episodes that upset them. Or they may voice general complaints that they or others have about the child. The specific episodes and general complaints are important to note, but they do not provide a differentiated picture of the child's competencies and problems. Nor do they tell the practitioner whether the child is really deviant or what the child's particular strengths and weaknesses are. By using the empirically based assessment forms early in the referral process, the practitioner obtains a more differentiated picture of the child than is typically conveyed by the referral complaints.

Most parents who have at least fifth-grade reading skills can independently fill out the CBCL/2-3 in 10 minutes and the CBCL/4-18 in 15 to 17 minutes. However, if it is unclear whether a parent or other informant can independently fill out the CBCL, we recommend that an interviewer hand the informant a copy of the form, saying, "I'll read you the questions on this form and I'll write down your answers." Informants who can read well enough will usually start answering the questions without waiting for them to be read, but this procedure avoids the embarrassment and errors incurred if an informant cannot read well. Even for informants who cannot read well, looking at the form provides them with the same view of the questions as provided to those who complete the form independently. For informants who do not know English, translations are available in some 50 languages (Brown & Achenbach, 1996, list the translations available at this writing).

Informants who fill out the form independently should be given opportunities to ask for clarification of items by a person familiar with the forms. If informants request clarification, their questions should be answered in a factual manner designed to help them describe the child's behavior as accurately as possible. Informants should also be encouraged to add comments as needed.

Because the empirically based forms sample diverse aspects of functioning, they can reveal competencies and problems that might be missed by interviews or instruments that focus only on a particular referral complaint, such as hyperactivity. Furthermore, the practitioner can use the completed forms as a takeoff point for interviewing. For example, if a parent has completed the CBCL, the practitioner can first ask whether the parent has any questions about the CBCL. The practitioner can also ask about the specific competencies, descriptions of problems, best things about the child, and concerns that the parent indicated on the CBCL. This procedure helps the practitioner obtain a quick picture of the parent's view of the child in many areas. The practitioner can thus save valuable interview time for tasks that are not amenable to standardization, such as evaluating the details of the child's living situation, contingencies that may affect the child's problem behavior, and the family's workability for various possible interventions.

Sequences for Gathering Data

Sequences for gathering data will vary according to the nature of individual cases, the settings in which they are seen, and the availability of relevant informants. Despite case-by-case variations, flowcharts can provide helpful reminders about when different empirically based procedures would typically be used and where they mesh with other data-gathering procedures. The flowchart in Figure 4.1 outlines a typical data-gathering sequence.

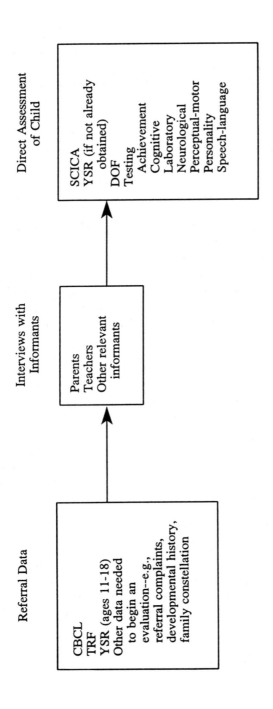

Referral Data

CBCL
TRF
YSR (ages 11-18)
Other data needed
   to begin an
   evaluation--e.g.,
referral complaints,
developmental history,
family constellation

Interviews with
Informants

Parents
Teachers
Other relevant
   informants

Direct Assessment
of Child

SCICA
YSR (if not already
      obtained)
DOF
Testing
   Achievement
   Cognitive
   Laboratory
   Neurological
   Perceptual-motor
   Personality
   Speech-language

Figure 4.1. Outline of typical data-gathering sequence.

85

Referral Data. The box labeled Referral Data on the left side of Figure 4.1 lists the CBCL, TRF, YSR, and other data typically needed to begin an evaluation. Depending on their setting, practitioners may request parents to complete the CBCL long enough before their first interview to allow the CBCL to be scored and the practitioner to review it in preparation for the first interview. This can be done by mailing CBCLs to parents prior to their first appointment and asking them to return the completed CBCLs by a date early enough to permit scoring before their first appointment.

In situations where parents do not mail in completed CBCLs, an alternative is to have parents come about 30 minutes before their interview to fill out the CBCL and have it scored in time for the practitioner to see before the interview. Several options are available to facilitate rapid scoring. One option is to have each parent complete the regular CBCL form and then to have a clerical worker key-enter the data into the scoring program, which is faster than using hand-scored profiles. A second option is to have each parent complete a machine-readable CBCL form and then have a clerical worker check the forms and feed them through an image scanner or a reflective-read scanner. Our Scanning Software Package is available for transmitting the data from the scanner to the scoring program for the CBCL. The same forms and scanning software can be used with data transmitted by fax. The software that reads CBCLs can also read TRFs and YSRs (Jacobowitz, 1996). A third is to have parents enter their CBCL data directly into a computer where our Client Entry Program transmits the data to the scoring program. The same Client Entry Program also enables teachers and youths to enter TRF and YSR data, respectively (Arnold, 1996). Table 4.1 summarizes these options for entering and scoring data. Even if it is not possible to have the CBCL scored before an interview, the completed CBCL can provide the practitioner with a takeoff point for interviewing, as outlined earlier.

Because parents typically need to provide demographic, background, and insurance information, they can do this while the CBCL is being scored. As indicated in Figure 4.1, it is desirable to obtain information on specific referral complaints, developmental history, and family constellation as early as possible. It may be convenient to obtain this information by having parents complete forms or by having a paraprofessional obtain the information from parents while the CBCL is being scored.

If a referral is initiated by a teacher, as often occurs for school-based evaluations, the TRF may be the initial empirically based assessment form. TRF forms completed by teachers can be key-entered into the

TABLE 4.1 Options for Obtaining and Scoring CBCL/4-18, TRF, and YSR Data

Obtaining Data	*Scoring Data*
1. Informant fills out classic forms using pencil or pen[a]	1. (a) Key entry into profile scoring program (b) Hand-scoring on profile forms
2. Informant fills out machine-readable "bubble" forms[a]	2. Scanning Software Package transmits data from fax or scanner to profile scoring program
3. Informant enters data into computer	3. Client-Entry Program transmits data to profile scoring program

NOTE: Information on forms and software can be obtained from: Child Behavior Checklist, 1 South Prospect Street, Burlington, VT 05401-3456. Fax: 802-656-2602.
a. For informants who have less than fifth-grade reading skills or are otherwise impaired, an interviewer can read the items aloud and fill out the form. When an interviewer reads aloud from one copy of the form, it is usually helpful for the informant to be looking at a second copy of the form.

profile scoring program or entered on hand-scoring profile forms. Machine-readable TRFs can save the labor of key entry or hand scoring. The Client Entry Program can also be used if teachers have access to a computer. Because the Client Entry Program can run on notebook computers, teachers can use notebook computers to enter the data at any convenient time and location.

In some settings, it may be feasible to obtain the YSR as part of the referral process. Examples include settings in which adolescents seek help for themselves and situations in which the adolescent is cooperating with parents or teachers in the referral process. The same options are available for obtaining and scoring YSR data as for CBCL and TRF data, as outlined in Table 4.1.

Interviewing Informants. Interviews with adult informants constitute an important part of most services to children, both to obtain assessment data and because the adults are responsible for obtaining the services. Parents and parent surrogates are usually among the first to be interviewed as part of the data-gathering process, but initial interviews may involve a complex mixture of agendas and emotions.

Parents are often under pressure from other people, such as teachers, to do something about their children's problems. Among parents who have not previously sought professional help for behavioral and emotional problems, there is often trepidation, guilt, and uncertainty about how they may have contributed to the problems, whether they will be blamed, and what will be expected of them. Conflicts between family members may complicate initial interviews if parents blame each other for the child's problems or blame the child for causing problems in the family. Interpersonal issues may also arise between parents and the practitioner as each party evaluates the other. Uncertainties about costs and other constraints on services can further complicate the initial contacts.

The multiple issues involved in initial interviews can make it hard to obtain accurate information about the child's functioning. If the practitioner uses empirically based assessment forms completed by parents as takeoff points for interviewing, this will contribute to a joint problem-solving attitude that can help to demystify the initial contacts between the practitioner and parents. After discussing the completed CBCLs with parents, the practitioner can move on to other issues that do not lend themselves to standardized assessment. Table 4.2 outlines components of a parent interview that are relevant to most cases, although the precise sequences and interpersonal issues would vary with the case and setting.

For children with school problems, it is often helpful to interview teachers, either by phone or in person. In such cases, most components of the parent interview shown in Table 4.2 can be adapted for teachers. Initial interviews with both parents and teachers should accomplish tasks such as the following:

1. To establish effective communication between the practitioner and the informants.
2. To create a sense of collaborative problem solving.
3. To obtain details of the child's history and current functioning as seen by each informant.
4. To assess each informant's effect on the child in terms of how the informant may help and/or hinder the child.
5. To determine what each informant has tried and may be capable of doing to help the child.
6. To lay groundwork for the next steps, which may include comprehensive evaluation of the case, consultations with parents or teachers, decisions about interventions, and implementation of interventions.

Directly Assessing the Child. In most cases, direct assessment of the child begins after referral data are obtained and initial interviews with one

TABLE 4.2 Components of a Parent Interview

I. Purpose and confidentiality

II. Details of presenting problems
   Discussion of parents' responses to CBCL
   Nature of specific behaviors (descriptions, frequency, duration)
   Antecedent, sequential, and consequent conditions
   Situational and temporal variation in behavior
   Parent's feelings about identified problems
   Parent's usual response to problems
   Parent's preferred behaviors

III. History related to problems
   Onset of identified problems
   Relevant developmental and medical history

IV. Other possible problem areas
   Other emotional and behavioral problems
   Educational performance (if not covered above)
   Child's social relationships
   Child's family relationships

V. Family factors and stressors
   Family composition and demographics
   Family stressors (environmental, financial, health, psychosocial)
   Psychiatric/psychological problems in family members
   Alcohol or drug abuse by family members
   Marital relationships/satisfaction

VI. Feasibility of interventions
   Parent's usual discipline and reward procedures
   Cooperation between parents in discipline and rewards
   Past and current treatment efforts (educational, mental health, social services)
   Parent's reactions to possible interventions
   Formulation of initial goals and intervention plans
   Appointments for further problem analysis and interventions, if needed

SOURCE: Adapted from McConaughy (1996). Reprinted with permission from PRO-ED.

or more adult informants are done. For ages 11 to 18, the YSR enables the practitioner to obtain self-reports in a format like that of the CBCL/4-18 and TRF. The cross-informant computer program, described in Chapter 2, makes direct comparisons of YSR item and scale scores with those obtained from other informants. The program also prints correlations that indicate the degree of agreement between the youth and other informants.

Whether the YSR is obtained as part of the referral data or later, it provides an exceptionally useful takeoff point for interviewing adolescents. In interviews, adolescents may be resistant, deny problems, or have difficulty discussing their problems even if they are motivated to do so. However, when adolescents complete the YSR, they may report problems, such as suicidal ideation, strange thoughts, or feelings of rejection, that might not be revealed in interviews.

When interviewing adolescents who have completed the YSR, practitioners can follow the procedure outlined earlier for interviewing parents who have completed the CBCL. After asking whether there are any questions about the YSR, the practitioner can ask the adolescent to elaborate on particular problems and comments indicated on the YSR. Some adolescents will spontaneously begin talking about problems they have indicated on the YSR. This provides the practitioner with a rich opportunity to forge a therapeutic alliance. On the other hand, some adolescents' YSRs will report far fewer problems than are reported on their parents' CBCLs and teachers' TRFs. If there is considerable consistency among multiple adults in reporting problems that are not reported on the YSR, the practitioner can probe to determine whether the adolescent is unaware of the problems or is aware of them but resists acknowledging them.

In addition to the YSR, empirically based direct assessment procedures include the SCICA. The observational and self-report items of the SCICA can be scored for ages 6 to 18. Syndrome scales have been derived for ages 6 to 12, and work is under way on scales for ages 13-18 (McConaughy & Achenbach, 1994b). Designed to serve as an initial interview that covers various aspects of functioning, the SCICA also includes questions about problems reported by the child's parents and teachers. The questions assess the child's readiness to acknowledge problems that are of concern to others.

Where there are major discrepancies between reports by different teachers or between reports by a teacher and parents, the DOF can play a crucial role in documenting a child's actual behavior in classrooms and other group settings. The documentation provided by the DOF includes a descriptive record of what the child does during the observational sessions, the behavior of others toward the child, on-task scores, and problem scale scores that can be compared with scores obtained by two "control" children observed in the same setting, as well as with a reference group of children observed in many schools (Achenbach, 1991b; McConaughy,

Achenbach, & Gent, 1988). All these kinds of data can be used to determine whether a child displays significant behavioral problems, what kinds of problems are displayed, and how deviant the child is, both in comparison to classmates and to a broader normative sample.

In addition to shedding light on discrepancies between reports by different informants, DOF findings can also contribute to decisions about eligibility for special education and about specific interventions. Observational data can be obtained at low cost by training teacher aides and other paraprofessionals to use the DOF.

Other Assessment Procedures. Ability and achievement tests are often needed to determine whether achievement is enough below ability to qualify for special education. Inclusion of two achievement subtests in the SCICA may obviate the need for more extensive testing, if the child performs well on the two subtests and no other questions about achievement or ability are raised. Personality tests and procedures designed to assess a single problem area such as hyperactivity (e.g., Conners, 1990), depression (e.g., Kovacs, 1981), or perceptual-motor functioning (e.g., Bender Gestalt Test; Koppitz, 1975) would be administered at the practitioner's discretion. In addition, standardized assessment of speech-language development may be needed in some cases (e.g., Clinical Evaluation of Language Fundamentals-Revised; Semel, Wiig, & Secord, 1987).

A child's medical history and physical condition should always be considered in comprehensive evaluations of behavioral and emotional problems. The history should include physical development, developmental milestones, major illnesses and injuries, past and current medications and their effects, and current medical status. If necessary, laboratory and neurological tests should be requested to evaluate possible physical abnormalities that may contribute to behavioral and emotional problems.

CASE FORMULATION

After obtaining assessment data, the practitioner should identify important similarities and differences among the findings, formulate a comprehensive picture of the case, and select targets for change as a basis for case management. Figure 4.2 outlines the steps that are typically involved in case formulations.

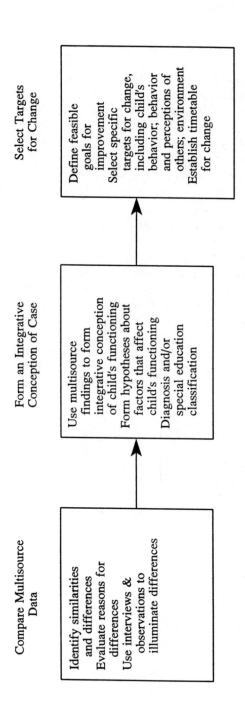

Figure 4.2. Illustrative components of case formulation.

Comparing Multisource Data

As indicated in the leftmost box of Figure 4.2, an initial step in case formulations is to identify similarities and differences in the picture of the child obtained from different sources. Where there are major differences between syndrome scores, profile patterns, or specific items scored from reports by parents versus teachers or from reports by different teachers, the DOF may shed light on the differences by documenting classroom behavior, as described earlier. If the DOF is not feasible or is not relevant to the obtained discrepancies, interviews with the informants may illuminate the discrepancies.

As an example, suppose that a mother's CBCL yields a high score on the Aggressive Behavior syndrome, because she assigned scores of 2 to many items such as *Physically attacks people*. Suppose, too, that the father's CBCL yielded a lower score on the Aggressive Behavior syndrome, because he scored the same items 0 or 1. If the parents are fairly sophisticated, the practitioner may elect to show them the contrasting profiles obtained from their CBCLs. If the parents are less sophisticated, it may be preferable to ask them about specific items. For example, the practitioner may ask the mother to describe the behavior on which she based her score of 2 for *Physically attacks people*. The practitioner can then ask the father if he had observed such behavior. It may thus be possible to determine the reasons for discrepancies in what the parents reported.

Perhaps both parents have observed the same behavior, but they either interpret it differently or differ in their candor about it. Or it may become evident that the behavior occurs only in the presence of one parent, because the parents' interactions with the child differ in ways that affect the behavior. Another possibility is that one parent is a poor informant, either because of selective or meager contact with the child or because that parent's reports are inaccurate, as judged from evidence for unfitness or major inconsistencies with everything else that is known about the child. Interviews may also be used to illuminate discrepancies between parent and teacher reports, as well as between reports by multiple teachers.

If the practitioner concludes that major discrepancies between different sources of data reflect true variations in the child's behavior, it may be possible to identify contingencies that explain the variations. For example, if aggressive behavior is evident only in the presence of one teacher, the behavior of that teacher or the context in which the child interacts with that teacher should be evaluated to determine what evokes the aggression and how it might be reduced. On the other hand, if scores for aggressive behavior are similarly high across multiple informants and aggressive behavior has persisted for a long time, this would indicate that more than situational contingencies are involved, as illustrated by the case of Kyle in Chapters 1 and 2.

Forming an Integrative Conception of the Case

As indicated in the middle box of Figure 4.2, the next step in the case formulation is to use the multisource findings to form an integrative conception of the case. That is, after evaluating similarities and differences in multisource data, the practitioner needs to apply clinical judgment and creativity to forming a mental representation of the case that highlights the important features of the child, family, school situation, and environment relevant to the child's functioning. The practitioner's conception of the case would usually involve hypotheses about how particular factors affect the child's functioning and about how each factor might be modified.

Based on an integrative conception of the case, the practitioner would decide whether criteria were met for particular *DSM* or *ICD* diagnoses and/or for particular categories of eligibility for special education, if such decisions are needed. As outlined later, elevated scores on some of the empirically based syndromes provide evidence to support particular *DSM* diagnoses and special education eligibilities.

To illustrate the relevance of conclusions drawn from multisource data, let us return to the example of deviance on the Aggressive Behavior syndrome that is specific to a particular informant or context versus aggressive behavior that is cross-situationally consistent and persistent. Evidence reviewed in Chapter 3 suggests that some individuals' aggression may have a traitlike quality that persists across developmental periods. The evidence also indicates that, although their socially intrusive behavior continues, some of these individuals show a reduction in physically aggressive behavior from adolescence to adulthood (Achenbach et al., 1995c). It is therefore possible that appropriate interventions can help at least some aggressive individuals channel the most harmful aspects of their behavior into less harmful forms. Such cases are especially challenging, because concerted cross-situational efforts are apt to be needed to rechannel their aggression. However, the harm done by persistent aggression, especially in adolescence and adulthood, warrants substantial efforts to reduce it. To form an integrative conception of a case involving deviance on the Aggressive Behavior syndrome, we would need to weigh issues of this sort.

Other kinds of problems may be less harmful and more tractable than those reflected in high scores on the Aggressive Behavior syndrome. However, similar principles apply to forming an integrative conception of the case. The integrative conception should take account of the particular mixtures of competencies and problems revealed by profiles scored from reports by different informants. For example, if a child is deviant only on the Attention Problems syndrome in CBCL, TRF, and YSR ratings, this would argue for interventions that are specific to ADHD, such as medication and classroom accommodations. On the other hand, if Attention Problems syndrome scores are elevated in ratings by multiple informants, but the Anxious/Depressed syndrome is also elevated in ratings by some informants and the Social Problems syndrome is elevated in ratings by other informants, this indicates a need to deal with dysphoric affect that may be occurring in some contexts and interpersonal problems in other contexts. Academic performance that is well below the child's ability level would also argue for remedial education, as reducing attention problems via medication alone is unlikely to compensate for deficits in other areas, even if the deficits initially resulted from attention problems.

Selecting Targets for Change

After constructing an integrative conception of the case on the basis of multisource data, the practitioner needs to select targets for change, as indicated in the rightmost box of Figure 4.2. This involves defining goals for improvement that are feasible, given the realities of the child's developmental level, competencies, family context, available resources, and efficacy of relevant intervention methods. As an example, for a child with good competencies whose behavior problems occur in one context and are evoked by contingencies in that context, those contingencies would be targeted for change. This might involve changing both the behavior of the child to avoid or respond differently to the problem situation and changing the behavior of others in the situation.

For cross-situationally consistent problems, the child's overall behavior pattern would be a more appropriate target for change. This might involve reducing stressors, strengthening competencies, and providing new incentives for the child, as well as replacing specific maladaptive behaviors with more adaptive ones. To accomplish such goals, it might be necessary to reduce marital conflict, improve parenting skills, protect a child from abuse, or modify a classroom environment rather than trying to change the child independently of these pathogenic influences. Because multiple factors are often involved, practitioners usually need to prioritize targets according to their judgment about the feasibility of change and the potential payoffs in terms of helping the child and providing stepping stones toward more advanced goals.

In addition to prioritizing targets for change, it is also important to establish a time table for achieving therapeutic goals. Financial constraints on the length of services are making timetables increasingly necessary. Yet, even without financial constraints, timetables are important for defining goals and encouraging continuous monitoring of progress. If goals are not met within reasonable periods, than the goals or means for achieving them may need changing.

CASE MANAGEMENT AND
OUTCOME EVALUATION

Implementing Interventions

Based on the case formulation and targets for change, the practitioner decides what interventions to implement, if any. Examples of interventions are listed in the leftmost box of Figure 4.3. Various combinations of these and other interventions should be selected according to evidence for their efficacy in ameliorating the problems that are targeted for change.

A large body of research has demonstrated the efficacy of a variety of interventions for childhood problems, especially for problems that were specifically targeted by the interventions (Weisz, Weiss, Han, Granger, & Morton, 1995). On the other hand, studies of children who received mental health services under more ordinary clinical conditions have not yielded much evidence for efficacy (Weisz, Donenberg, Han, & Kauneckis, 1995).

The greater efficacy of interventions in research contexts appears attributable to the following factors: (a) greater use of behavioral and cognitive-behavioral methods in the research contexts than under ordinary clinical conditions; (b) use of methods that focused more specifically on the target problems in the research contexts than under ordinary clinical conditions; and (c) use of more structured intervention procedures that fostered greater adherence to treatment plans in the research contexts than under ordinary clinical conditions (Weisz, Donenberg, et al., 1995). All

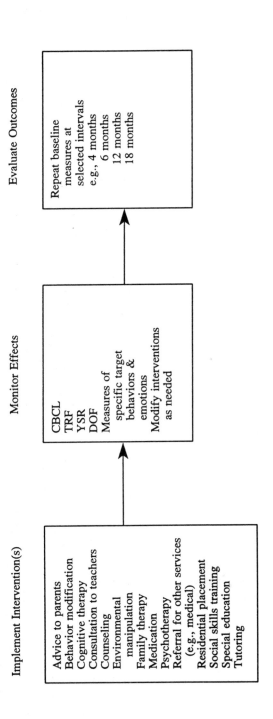

Figure 4.3. Illustrative components of case management and outcome evaluation.

these factors can potentially be applied to improving the efficacy of interventions under most clinical conditions. Consequently, by consulting sources such as Kendall and Panichelli-Mindel (1995) and Weisz, Weiss, et al. (1995) for interventions that have worked with particular kinds of problems, practitioners can maximize efficacy by matching intervention methods to specific problems and by adhering closely to treatment plans.

Monitoring Effects

To maximize the efficacy of interventions, we need to monitor changes in the target problems and competencies. As indicated in the middle box of Figure 4.3, the empirically based assessment forms and other procedures that are initially used to evaluate the child can be readministered after interventions have had time to take effect. More specialized monitoring of specific target problems and competencies may also be helpful, such as tabulations of specific behaviors, diary records of child and parent behavior, and use of narrowly focused scales, such as those designed to measure depression or hyperactivity. However, monitoring should not be confined only to the target problems and competencies, because important changes for better or worse may occur in other areas, as well. For example, if attention problems are identified as the main target for treatment, reassessments that focus only on attention problems may miss changes in other areas, such as dysphoric affect, which sometimes occurs when stimulant medications are used to treat attention problems.

By readministering the CBCL, TRF, and/or YSR to the informants who completed them initially, the practitioner can determine whether similar changes are evident in reports by all informants or whether cross-informant variations suggest that interventions are not having consistent effects. For instruments that specify a particular base rating period, such as 6 months for the problem items on the CBCL/4-18, the instructions to informants should be changed to be consistent with the period when interventions are presumed to have taken effect and should not overlap with the period covered by the initial ratings. For example, if the CBCL is to be readministered 4 months after it was initially completed by a parent, the parent should be asked to base ratings on a period of less than 4 months to avoid overlap with the initial rating period. Because the baseline rating period for the TRF is 2 months and because the DOF assesses particular 10-minute samples of behavior, these instruments would not require any adjustments when used to monitor the effects of interventions.

Evaluating Outcomes

Outcome findings have been published from research on numerous interventions for childhood problems (e.g., Weisz, Weiss, et al., 1995). However, the growth of managed care is greatly increasing demands for outcome evaluations of clinical case management. One kind of demand stems from needs by competing managed care organizations to provide prospective clients with evidence for the efficacy of their services. Another kind of demand stems from managed care organizations' needs to determine which interventions are most cost-effective within their own services. A third kind of demand stems from the needs of individual practitioners to determine whether interventions have ameliorated problems without continuing services longer than necessary and to document outcomes for purposes of quality assurance.

As indicated in Figure 4.3, outcomes can be evaluated by repeating procedures that were used to assess a child's baseline problems and competencies before intervention. In some respects, outcome evaluations can be viewed as continuations of the reassessments that would be done when monitoring effects to determine whether interventions should be modified. However, conclusions can be more effectively generalized across cases if uniform procedures and intervals are used to evaluate outcomes than if the procedures vary from case-to-case, as may be appropriate for monitoring individual children. It is therefore useful to select an interval between the initial assessment and first outcome assessment that can be applied fairly uniformly to most cases seen in a particular setting. For example, if interventions in a setting do not usually exceed 2 months, outcome assessments can be uniformly scheduled at 4 months after the initial assessment. If interventions may last up to 4 months, 6-month outcome assessments would be appropriate.

To avoid confounding with effects that are associated with termination, outcome assessments should be scheduled at least 1 month after termination. It is also desirable to have additional outcome assessments, such as at 12 and 18 months after the initial assessment, to evaluate longer-term outcomes. By using the empirically based assessment forms, practitioners can conduct outcome assessments by having clerical personnel mail the forms to parents, teachers, and/or youths at the scheduled intervals. If informants fail to return completed forms, they can be asked to respond to the assessment questions by phone.

Because T scores, percentiles, and normal ranges are provided for the empirically based scales, clinically significant improvements can be inferred from scale scores that have moved from the clinical to the normal range, as recommended by Jacobson and Truax (1991). The magnitude of change can also be judged by comparing the T scores on each scale before versus after an intervention. If the same procedures are used for initial and outcome assessments over uniform intervals for substantial numbers of children, statistical analyses can be used to test the statistical significance of changes. Statistical analyses can also be used to determine whether outcomes are significantly better for children who received particular interventions than for other children.

APPLICATIONS IN
PARTICULAR CONTEXTS

The foregoing sections provided an overview of how empirically based assessment procedures can generally be used. It is also important to note some variations that are appropriate for particular contexts, as outlined in the following sections.

Managed Care Contexts

The numerous contemporary approaches to managed care are greatly complicating mental health services for children. On the other hand, the principles of managed care offer opportunities for improving services by making efficiency and efficacy more important than maximum reimbursability, which tends to drive practices under the traditional fee-for-service system. The importance of efficiency and efficacy is especially evident under capitated managed care, where an organization receives a fixed annual payment (capitation) for providing services to each member.

When an organization receives a capitation for each member and must compete with other organizations for members, it has economic incentives to be well-informed about the problems of its members, to closely monitor relations between its members' problems and the services provided, and to determine which services keep members healthy and satisfied at minimal cost. To survive over the long run, organizations must continually use information to improve services. This necessitates investment in information technology that can monitor members' problems from the beginning of service contacts to the evaluation of outcomes.

In well-structured organizations, it is economical to invest in technology and personnel to obtain standardized data that will improve decision-making and make services more cost-effective. For example, in settings where many children are seen for mental health or pediatric services, it may be cost-effective to invest in scanning equipment that can quickly process large numbers of assessment forms, as well as other forms needed by the organization. Scanning equipment makes it possible to quickly and cheaply provide profiles scored from machine-readable CBCLs, TRFs, and YSRs to practitioners, who can then use them according to the flowchart in Figure 4.1. Thereafter, the same personnel who initially obtain the completed forms can obtain and process reassessment forms to monitor the effects of interventions and to evaluate outcomes. In some settings, direct entry of data by parents and youths using the Client Entry Program may also be a cost-effective way to obtain data.

Managed care seeks to minimize the most expensive kinds of services, especially hospitalization. By periodically reassessing referred children to monitor the effects of interventions and to evaluate outcomes, practitioners can detect significant increases in problems that would warrant increased outpatient efforts to prevent hospitalization. If hospitalization is nevertheless necessary, a standardized database that documents the course of the child's problems and competencies prior to hospitalization can be helpful in selecting appropriate goals for hospitalization. For example, if a child shows large increases in scores on the Anxious/Depressed, Withdrawn, and Thought Problems syndromes in response to major stresses, a day treatment program designed to help the child cope with the stresses might be more therapeutic at lower cost than full-time hospitalization. Periodic reassessments using the empirically based procedures can indicate whether the selected treatment is then followed by increases in competencies and decreases in problems. Continued use of the same assessment procedures also facilitates the design and monitoring of aftercare to ensure that it will prevent relapses.

Carve-Outs of Mental Health Services. Much of the foregoing scenario is consistent with how well-structured managed care organizations provide some of their services and how managed mental health services can potentially be provided. However, some managed care firms structure mental health care quite differently from other health care. Sometimes referred to as "carve-outs," the different ways of structuring mental health care often involve more restrictive gatekeeping mechanisms for mental health services than for medical services. As an example, mental health services are often subject to deductible and co-pay requirements, restrictions on the number of sessions, and limits on hospitalization that do not apply to medical services. Furthermore, many managed care plans require advance authorization for mental health services, and practitioners are required to repeatedly document the target problems and treatment. The restrictive approach to mental health services is understandable in light of several differences from medical services for physical illnesses. One difference is that physical illnesses usually involve abnormalities or dysfunctions that can be documented more unambiguously than can most behavioral and emotional problems. A second difference is that mental health services span a wide range of philosophies, practitioners, and methods for which there is less consensus and less systematic outcome evidence than for many treatments of physical illnesses. And a third difference is that some individuals are heavy users of costly mental health services in the absence of evidence that they have problems that will benefit from such services.

To overcome discrimination against mental health services, it is necessary to advance assessment of problems, the application of effective interventions, and outcome evaluations that demonstrate improvement at reasonable cost. As illustrated throughout this book, empirically based assessment is designed to facilitate all these efforts. However, to ensure that mental health services are adequately supported by managed care, it is necessary for mental health practitioners and researchers to overcome the ambiguities that lead to discriminatory carve-outs.

Fee-for-Service Contexts

Despite the growth of managed care, many practitioners continue to work at least partly under fee-for-service conditions. The tendency of managed care plans to carve out mental health services by contracting with independent practitioners is maintaining one variant of the fee-for-service model, although usually at lower fees and under more restrictive conditions than practitioners desire. Indemnity insurance companies, Medicaid, and public agencies also continue to pay practitioners on a fee-for-service basis, although many of these payers are adopting managed care methods to control mental health services. Regardless of the future course of managed care, however, a market will likely remain for fee-for-service care that is paid for by those able to afford it.

Whereas efficiency and efficacy have high priority within managed care organizations, fee-for-service arrangements have been dependent on *DSM* and *ICD* diagnoses as a basis for payment. With respect to childhood disorders, some third-party payers do not cover services for some diagnoses, such as ODD. Others do not cover certain types of treatment for certain diagnoses.

The use of diagnoses to determine reimbursement has greatly increased practitioners' attention to diagnosis. Although *DSM* diagnoses are the most widely publicized in the United States, mental health services within medical settings and some insurance companies require *ICD* diagnoses, because the *ICD* is the official system for coding diseases in the United States, as well as in most other countries. *DSM-IV* (pp. 829-841) lists relations between its diagnostic categories and *ICD* codes. However, there are many differences between the two systems in the names they provide for their childhood diagnoses, in the descriptions and criteria for the diagnoses, and in multiaxial aspects of the systems. Practitioners who are familiar with the *DSM* system must therefore make adjustments when they need to provide third-party payers with *ICD* diagnoses.

Because the empirically based approach quantifies aggregations of problems according to their patterns of co-occurrence, it does not necessarily yield findings that can be directly translated into either *DSM* or *ICD* diagnoses. Nevertheless, as summarized in Chapter 3, numerous studies have found statistically significant associations between *DSM* diagnoses and scores on the empirically based syndromes. The changes from *DSM-III* and *DSM-III-R* to *DSM-IV* leave open the question of how strongly *DSM-IV* diagnoses will agree with either the diagnoses based on the earlier editions of the *DSM* or with scores on the empirically based syndromes. However, Table 4.3 lists descriptive relations between *DSM-IV* diagnostic categories and the cross-informant syndromes. High scores on the syndromes listed in the right-hand column of Table 4.3 reflect the kinds of problems represented by the *DSM-IV* diagnoses listed in the left-hand column.

Mental health services in fee-for-service contexts may be customized to a greater extent than in managed care organizations, where certain assessment and service procedures are likely to be applied uniformly to most cases. Flexibility to vary assessment procedures is enhanced by the multiple options for processing the CBCL/4-18, TRF, and YSR, including hand scoring, key entry, client entry, fax, and scanning. Because practitioners, paraprofessionals, and clerical workers can obtain scored profiles by any of these methods, no specialized personnel are needed.

Whichever combination of assessment procedures the practitioner chooses, the forms completed by informants and the profiles scored from them can provide low cost documentation of the child's pretreatment functioning, as seen by each informant. By having informants complete

TABLE 4.3　Approximate Relations Between *DSM-IV* Disorders and
Empirically Based Syndromes

DSM-IV Disorder	CBCL/TRF/YSR
Attention-Deficit/Hyperactivity	Attention Problems
Conduct	Aggressive Behavior
	Delinquent Behavior
Dysthymic	Anxious/Depressed
Generalized Anxiety	Anxious/Depressed
Major Depressive	Anxious/Depressed
Oppositional Defiant	Aggressive Behavior
Somatization	Somatic Complaints
Undifferentiated Somatoform	Somatic Complaints

the forms again after treatment, the practitioner can document changes and determine whether further treatment is needed. The pre- and posttreatment profiles can also be used to support claims for reimbursement from third-party payers, if necessary. In addition, because the SCICA is designed to obtain the kinds of data and impressions usually sought in clinical evaluation interviews, it can be used as the initial interview with the child, thereby providing standardized documentation for the direct assessment conducted by the practitioner.

School Contexts

The Individuals with Disabilities Education Act (IDEA; Public Law 101-476, 1990) requires schools to provide special education services for children with disabilities. The empirically based assessment procedures are especially helpful for determining whether children qualify for special education under the IDEA category of Serious Emotional Disturbance (SED), which is defined as follows:

(i) The term means a condition exhibiting one or more of the following characteristics over a long period of time and to a marked degree, which adversely affects educational performance:

A. An inability to learn which cannot be explained by intellectual, sensory, or other health factors;

B. An inability to build or maintain satisfactory interpersonal relationships with peers and teachers;

C. Inappropriate types of behavior or feelings under normal circumstances;

D. A general pervasive mood of unhappiness or depression; or

E. A tendency to develop physical symptoms or fears associated with
personal or school problems;

(ii) The term includes children who are schizophrenic. The term does not
include children who are socially maladjusted unless it is determined
that they have a serious emotional disturbance.

Table 4.4 outlines relations between the IDEA criteria for SED and the
empirically based syndromes that most clearly assess each criterial feature. Table 4.4 also indicates how the assessment instruments can help
practitioners judge whether a child's disability exists over a long period
of time, is exhibited to a marked degree, and adversely affects educational
performance.

Schools can employ empirically based assessment by having teachers
complete the TRF for children referred for evaluation. By looking at the
profile scored from the TRF, the school psychologist or other practitioner
can quickly determine whether the problems reported by the teacher
actually exceed the normal range for the pupil's gender and age. If so, this
would argue for a more comprehensive evaluation that may include
CBCLs completed by the pupil's parents, the DOF to compare the pupil's
classroom behavior with the behavior of classmates and with the DOF
norms, and possibly the SCICA and YSR.

Cross-informant findings on scales relevant to the SED criteria would
be considered with other findings reviewed by a multidisciplinary team
(MDT) to determine eligibility for special education according to IDEA
criteria. The results of the empirically based procedures would also
provide data on which to base specific interventions. That is, the areas in
which the child was found to be deviant would be targeted for interventions. By periodically readministering the CBCL, TRF, DOF, and/or YSR,
school psychologists and special educators can determine whether pupils
are improving or whether interventions need to be modified.

Because schools are responsible for pupils over long periods of time,
it is in the best interest of the pupils and schools to try to ameliorate
significant problems, even among pupils who do not qualify for special
education under the IDEA criteria. For example, it may be cost-effective

TABLE 4.4 Relations Between IDEA Criteria for SED and Empirically Based Syndromes

IDEA Criteria for SED	CBCL, TRF, & YSR	SCICA	DOF
Inability to learn	Attention Problems	Attention Problems	Withdrawn-Inattentive
Inability to build or maintain relationships	Social Problems Withdrawn	Withdrawn	
Inappropriate types of behavior or feelings	Aggressive Behavior Thought Problems	Aggressive Behavior Resistant Strange	Nervous-Obsessive Attention-Demanding Aggressive, Hyperactive
General unhappiness	Anxious/Depressed	Anxious/Depressed	Depressed
Tendency to develop physical symptoms or fears	Anxious/Depressed Somatic Complaints	Anxious Anxious/Depressed	
Long period to time	Follow-up evaluations	Follow-up evaluations	Follow-up evaluations
Marked degree	High scores for total problems, Internalizing, Externalizing, or syndromes	High scores for total Observations, total Self-Reports, Internalizing, Externalizing, or syndromes	High scores for total problems, Internalizing, Externalizing, or syndromes
Adversely affects educational performance	Low scores for CBCL School, TRF Academic Performance, and/or TRF Adaptive Functioning	Low SCICA achievement test scores	Low on-task score

NOTE: Unfamiliar acronyms can be found in the List of Acronyms at the front of this book.

to obtain the TRF and/or the DOF for "at risk" pupils at regular intervals, such as every 4 months, to determine whether adjustments should be made in their school environments. Because many school systems have fax or scanning equipment to use for other purposes, machine-readable TRFs offer an efficient means for assessing referrals from teachers, as well as for periodic reassessments.

Forensic Contexts

Divorce and custody issues, juvenile delinquency, child abuse, and foster placements require practitioners to deal with forensic matters. When practitioners provide services that involve testifying in court or submitting reports for forensic purposes, they must document their findings in ways that go beyond subjective opinions based on unstandardized interviews. By obtaining empirically based assessment forms from multiple informants, such as a child's teachers, parents, and/or foster parents, the practitioner can submit findings that include comparisons between profiles scored from the different informants. If multiple informants indicate deviance on the same syndromes, this is apt to carry considerably more weight than a practitioner's subjective judgment.

By using the SCICA, the practitioner can compare interview data with data obtained from other instruments to demonstrate ways in which the interview either supports or contradicts other sources. Where the fitness or veracity of a particular informant is in question, such as a parent who is under suspicion, the profile scored from that informant's report can be compared with profiles scored from other informants' reports. If the informant who is in question reports far more, far fewer, or very different problems or competencies than the other informants, this would support suspicions about the informant's fitness or veracity. On the other hand, if the cross-informant computer program yields high correlations between the informant's scores and scores obtained from other informants, this would argue against such suspicions.

Periodic reevaluations of children for forensic purposes can also make use of the empirically based assessment procedures. For example, if a child is placed with one parent for a trial period in a disputed custody case, periodic reassessments that employ the TRF, SCICA, and/or YSR can be used to evaluate changes in the child's functioning independent of the parent's own reports. The effects of foster placements can also be evaluated by periodically obtaining empirically based assessment data from sources other than the foster parents, although CBCLs completed by the foster parents may be used to determine how well their reports agree with other data.

SUMMARY

This chapter provided an overview of how empirically based assessment is used in various contexts. By using the empirically based assessment forms early in the referral process, the practitioner can obtain a more differentiated picture of the child's competencies and problems than would be afforded by referral complaints. The empirically based forms can also be used as takeoff points for interviewing, enabling practitioners to reserve valuable interview time for aspects of assessment that need to be tailored to each case.

As part of the case formulation, the practitioner should compare multi-source data, construct an integrative conception of the case, and select targets for change in preparation for case management. Case management typically includes implementing interventions, monitoring the effects of interventions, and evaluating outcomes.

In managed care contexts that emphasize cost-effectiveness, efficiency, and efficacy, it is economical to invest in technology and personnel to obtain standardized data as a basis for decision making. In such contexts, scanning equipment may be particularly cost-effective for processing assessment forms obtained at referral, during the course of services, and for outcome evaluations. Empirically based assessment can be especially helpful in meeting the goals of capitated managed care systems, but it can also help to avoid discriminatory carve-outs.

In fee-for-service contexts, practitioners may customize their assessment procedures more than in managed care contexts, but empirically based assessment can improve their evaluation and case management procedures, as well as providing documentation for third-party reimbursement.

Special education laws require schools to clearly document the problems of pupils who are not functioning well. The empirically based procedures provide documentation for determining eligibility for special education services, for identifying specific targets for intervention, and for periodically reevaluating pupils' problems.

When dealing with forensic issues, practitioners can use empirically based assessment procedures to provide more persuasive evidence about children's functioning than is provided by subjective impressions from unstandardized interviews. The empirically based procedures can also be used to document children's functioning under various placement conditions, such as with a parent when custody is in question and with foster parents.

5

CASE ILLUSTRATIONS FOR
ELEMENTARY SCHOOL AGES

Our case illustrations include the five assessment axes outlined in Table 2.1. Our main focus is on parent reports, teacher reports, and direct assessment of the child to illustrate applications and interpretations of the empirically based instruments. Relevant information from cognitive and physical assessment is summarized. After presenting data for the five assessment axes, we render a case formulation based on integration of data obtained from multiple sources. Interventions are then described for each case, although these are not necessarily the only appropriate interventions. Follow-up assessments are also discussed to illustrate applications of the empirically based procedures to outcome evaluations.

This chapter illustrates empirically based assessment of 7-year-old Lonnie and 10-year-old Natalie. Chapters 1 and 2 introduced 12-year-old Kyle, whom we will meet again at age 15 in Chapter 6, along with 14-year-old Julie. These four cases exemplify a variety of problems, as reflected in the empirically based syndromes discussed in Chapters 2 and 3. Chapter 7 will present additional cases illustrating special assessment issues, including behavioral problems associated with mental retardation and a classwide intervention for first-grade children.

CASE 2. LONNIE:
A BOY WITH ATTENTION
AND SOCIAL PROBLEMS
(continued from Chapter 2)

Lonnie Parker, a cute, freckle-faced 7-year-old, was introduced in Chapter 2 when we presented the DOF. Lonnie was referred for evaluation of his disruptive behavior and learning problems, after being retained in first grade because of social immaturity. His previous first-grade teacher had complained that he took forever to get anything done and was boisterous and noisy. Lonnie's current teacher voiced similar concerns that he was disruptive in class and failed to complete assigned work.

Lonnie's mother agreed that he was an active child but thought this was typical of boys his age. She suspected that the teacher didn't like Lonnie and had trouble with him because she was young and inexperienced. She also doubted that Lonnie understood his assignments, because her attempts to help him with homework often led to tears and arguments. When he was home, Lonnie seemed like any happy 7-year-old. He spent much of his free time riding his bike with friends, but he could also spend hours drawing by himself when friends were not around.

After several phone calls from the teacher, Mrs. Parker started to worry that Lonnie's second year in first grade would be no better than his first year. The teacher urged her to seek medication for hyperactivity, but she was reluctant to do this. Instead, she agreed to a comprehensive evaluation by the school psychologist and special education staff. The evaluation included parent and teacher ratings on empirically based measures, parent and teacher interviews, standardized tests of Lonnie's cognitive ability and achievement, an interview with Lonnie, and direct observations in the classroom.

Parent Reports

Prior to meeting with the school psychologist, Mrs. Parker completed the CBCL/4-18. Her ratings produced scores in the normal range on the Activities, Social, and total competence scales, but a score in the borderline range on the School scale. Mrs. Parker reported that her son had two or three friends whom he saw regularly outside of school. She also listed interests in several activities and hobbies and participation in team sports and Sunday school. The CBCL/4-18 competence scores thus indicated normal social involvement but rather low school performance.

Figure 5.1 (pp. 112-113) shows Lonnie's scores on the CBCL/4-18 problem scales. Lonnie scored in the clinical range for total problems and in the borderline range for Internalizing, but in the normal range for Externalizing. On the syndrome scales, Lonnie showed marked peaks for Social Problems and Attention Problems. Lonnie's mother rated him 1 or 2 on six of the eight Social Problems items, such as *Acts too young for his age, Clings to adults or too dependent,* and *Doesn't get along with other children.* She also rated him 1 or 2 on seven of the eleven Attention

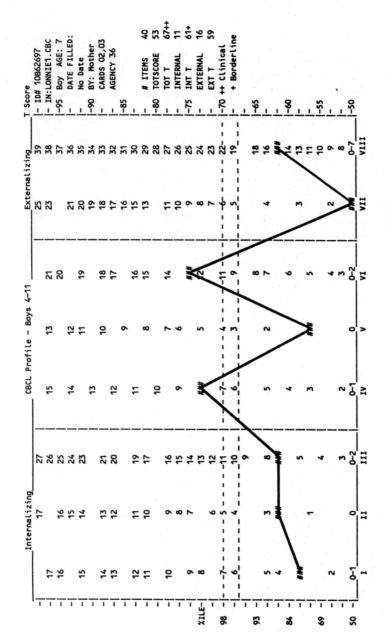

Figure 5.1. CBCL problem profile for Lonnie at age 7.

WITHDRAWN		SOMATIC COMPLAINTS		ANXIOUS/ DEPRESSED		SOCIAL PROBLEMS		THOUGHT PROBLEMS		ATTENTION PROBLEMS		DELINQUENT BEHAVIOR		AGGRESSIVE BEHAVIOR		OTHER PROBS	
1	42.Rather BeAlone	0	51. Dizzy	2	12.Lonely	2	1. Acts Young	0	9. Mind Off	2	1. Acts Young	1	26.NoGuilt	2	3. Argues	1	5. ActoppSex$
0	65.Won't Talk	0	54. Tired	0	14.Cries	1	11.Clings	0	40.Hears Things	2	8. Concen- trate	0	39.BadCompan	0	7. Brags	0	6. BM Out
0	69.Secret- ive	0	56a.Aches	1	31.FearDoBad	1	25.NotGet Along	0	66.Repeats Acts	2	10.Sit Still	0	43.LieCheat	0	16.Mean	0	15.CruelAnim
		1	56b.Head- aches	0	32.Perfect	1	38.Teased	0	70.Sees Things	2	13.Confuse	0	63.PrefOlder	1	19.DemAttn	0	18.HarmSelf
0	75.Shy	0	56c.Nausea	1	33.Unloved	1	48.Not Liked	0	80.Stares*	2	17.Day- dream	0	67.RunAway	1	20.DestOwn	1	24.NotEat
0	80.Stares	1	56d.Eye	2	34.OutToGet	0	55.Over- Weight*	1	84.Strange Behav	2	41.Impulsv	0	72.SetFires	0	21.DestOthr	0	28.EatNonFood
1	88.Sulks	0	56e.Skin	1	35.Worthless	0	62.Clumsy	0	85.Strange Ideas	0	45.Nervous	0	81.StealHome	1	22.DisbHome*	0	29.Fears
1	102.Under- active	0	56f.Stomach	0	45.Nervous	2	64.Prefers Young			0	46.Twitch*	0	82.StealOut	1	23.DisbSchl	0	30.FearSchool
0	103.Sad	0	56g.Vomit	0	50.Fearful					1	61.Poor School	0	90.Swears	0	27.Jealous	0	36.GetHurt
0	111.With- drawn			0	52.Guilty					0	62.Clumsy	1	96.ThinkSex*$	1	37.Fights	0	44.BiteNail
				0	71.SelfConsc					0	80.Stares	0	101.Truant	0	57.Attacks	0	47.Nightmares
				0	89.Suspic							0	105.AlcDrugs	0	68.Screams	0	49.Constipate
				0	103.Sad							0	106.Vandal*	2	74.ShowOff	0	53.Overeat
				0	112.Worries									1	86.Stubborn	0	56h.OtherPhys
														1	87.MoodChng	0	58.PickSkin
														2	93.TalkMuch	1	59.SexPrtsP$
														0	94.Teases	0	60.SexPrtsM$
														1	95.Temper	0	73.SexProbs$
														0	97.Threaten	0	76.SleepLess
														0	104.Loud	0	77.SleepMore
3	TOTAL	2	TOTAL	6	TOTAL	8	TOTAL	1	TOTAL	13	TOTAL	1	TOTAL	15	TOTAL	0	78.SmearBM
58	T SCORE	61	T SCORE	61	T SCORE	73	T SCORE	57	T SCORE	75	T SCORE	50	T SCORE	62	T SCORE	0	79.SpeechProb
44	CLIN T	49	CLIN T	44	CLIN T	59	CLIN T	44	CLIN T	59	CLIN T	38	CLIN T	44	CLIN T	2	83.StoresUp
																0	91.TalkSuicid
																0	92.SleepWalk
																1	98.ThumbSuck
																0	99.TooNeat
																0	100.SleepProb
																0	107.WetsSelf
																0	108.WetsBed
																1	109.Whining
																0	110.WshopSex$
																-	113.OtherProb

```
                       IX
                  SEX PROBLEMS
               1  TOTAL SCORE
              65  T SCORE
              $=Item on Sex
                 Probs Syndrome
```

*Items not on Cross-Informant Construct

Not in Total Problem Score
1 2.Allergy   0 4.Asthma

Profile Type:	WTHDR	SOMAT	SOCIAL	DEL-AGG	W-A/D-Agg	Delinq
ICC:	-.376	-.028	.392	-.309	-.316	-.436

No ICCs are significant

Figure 5.1. (Continued)

Problems items, including *Can't concentrate; Can't pay attention for long, Can't sit still, restless, or hyperactive;* and *Impulsive or acts without thinking.* Lonnie's scores on all other CBCL/4-18 scales were in the normal range.

Because Lonnie's teacher had expressed particular concerns about hyperactivity, she and Mrs. Parker were asked to complete the relevant versions of the Conners (1990) Rating Scales. The Conners Parent Rating Scale (CPRS) contains 48 problem items rated by parents on 4-point scales. Scores are provided for Conduct Problems, Learning Problems, Psychosomatic Problems, Impulsivity-Hyperactivity, and Anxiety, and there is a Hyperactivity Index. The CPRS for Lonnie produced clinical range scores for Learning Problems, Impulsivity-Hyperactivity, and the Hyperactivity Index.

In an interview with the school psychologist, Mrs. Parker discussed Lonnie's developmental history, as well as her strategies for coping with the problems revealed on the CBCL/4-18 and CPRS. The youngest of two children, Lonnie was the result of an unplanned pregnancy, which added to marital stress between his parents. The marriage ended in divorce when Lonnie was 2 years old. Lonnie's father, who maintained his own retail business, continued to visit regularly with the children every other weekend. Lonnie's mother began work as a legal secretary when Lonnie entered first grade. Prior to that time, she had done volunteer work in her daughter's classroom.

Mrs. Parker described Lonnie as "a bit of a rascal with a good sense of humor." He was a great talker, she said. He loved to tell jokes and stories and play pranks on his friends and his sister. He also clowned around at dinner and made odd noises in church. Although he showed normal development, except for slowness in learning to tie shoes, Lonnie seemed somewhat moody, was easily frustrated, and was quite active as a young child. He always wanted to do things his own way. However, he depended on his older sister to do many things for him, like tying his shoes, packing his lunch box, and picking up toys. He refused to do any schoolwork unless his mother or sister sat next to him to help. Lonnie did not seem hyperactive in preschool, according to his mother, but he did have trouble obeying rules. Shortly after he entered first grade, his teacher complained about his restlessness and refusal to work. By the end of first grade, he had failed to complete the necessary workbooks in reading and math. This led to a decision to retain him in first grade for the following year. When asked about discipline tactics, Mrs. Parker reported that she often scolded him and occasionally spanked him when he talked back or disobeyed rules. She sometimes sent him to his room. Lonnie's dawdling in the morning was especially frustrating as Mrs. Parker tried to get both children ready for school and leave for her job on time.

In addition to discussing Lonnie's developmental history and current problems, the school psychologist asked about symptoms for several *DSM-IV* psychiatric disorders. Mrs. Parker reported more than six of the nine symptoms of inattention and more than six of the nine symptoms of hyperactivity-impulsivity that are listed for the diagnosis of ADHD. Based on Mrs. Parker's reports, the school psychologist decided that Lonnie also met the ADHD criteria regarding onset, duration, and impairment.

Teacher Reports

On the TRF, Lonnie's current first-grade teacher rated his school performance as somewhat below grade level in reading, writing, and math, producing a score in the borderline range for academic performance. The teacher's ratings of adaptive functioning produced a score in the clinical range, reflecting ratings far below other pupils for how hard Lonnie was working and how appropriately he was behaving.

On the TRF problem scales, Lonnie scored in the clinical range for total problems and Externalizing and in the borderline range for Internalizing. Lonnie's profile showed peaks in the clinical range for Attention Problems and Aggressive Behavior, as illustrated in Figure 5.2 (pp. 116-117). Lonnie's teacher endorsed 19 of the 20 Attention Problems items, producing a very high score ($T = 86$) compared to the normative sample. The teacher endorsed many of the same items on this scale as did Lonnie's mother, plus additional items relevant to the school setting, such as *Difficulty following directions* and *Fails to carry out assigned tasks*. Lonnie's teacher also endorsed 23 of the 25 Aggressive Behavior items, including *Argues a lot, Demands a lot of attention, Disturbs other pupils, Disrupts class discipline, Gets in many fights,* and *Talks too much.* Lonnie's high score on the TRF Aggressive Behavior syndrome contrasted with a much lower score on the CBCL/4-18 version of this syndrome, indicating many more aggressive problems at school than at home. Lonnie's teacher scored him in the borderline range for Social Problems but in the normal range on the other TRF syndrome scales. An intraclass correlation (ICC) of .477 indicated that Lonnie's overall pattern of problems correlated significantly with the TRF Delinquent-Aggressive profile type.

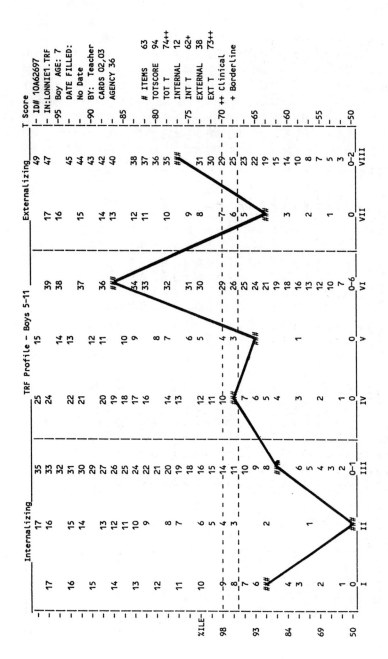

Figure 5.2. TRF problem profile for Lonnie at age 7.

WITHDRAWN	SOMATIC COMPLAINTS	ANXIOUS/ DEPRESSED	SOCIAL PROBLEMS	THOUGHT PROBLEMS	ATTENTION PROBLEMS	DELINQUENT BEHAVIOR	AGGRESSIVE BEHAVIOR	OTHER PROBS
0 42.Rather BeAlone	0 51. Dizzy	0 12.Lonely	2 1. Acts Young	1 9. Mind Off	2 1. Acts Young	1 26.NoGuilt	2 3. Argues	0 5. ActoppSex
0 65.Won't Talk	0 54. Tired	0 14.Cries	1 11.Clings	0 18.Harms Self*	2 2. Hums*	2 39.Bad Compan	1 6. Defiant*	0 28.EatNonFood
0 69.Secret- ive	0 56a.Aches	0 31.FearDoBad	0 12.Lonely*	0 29.Fears*	1 4. Finish*	0 43.LieCheat	1 7. Brags	0 30.FearSchool
0 75.Shy	0 56b.Head- aches	1 32.Perfect	0 14.Cries*	0 40.Hears Things	2 8.Concentr	0 63.Prefers Older	1 16.Mean	2 44.BiteNail
2 80.Stares	0 56c.Nausea	0 33.Unloved	1 25.NotGet Along	1 66.Repeats Acts	2 10.SitStil	0 82.Steals	2 19.DemAttn	2 46.Twitch
1 88.Sulks	0 56d.Eye	0 34.OutToGet	0 33.Unlove*	0 70.Sees Things	2 13.Confuse	0 90.Swears	1 20.DestOwn	0 55.Overweight
2 102.Under- active	0 56e.Skin	1 35.Worthless	0 34.OutTo Get*	0 84.Strange Behav	2 15.Fidget*	0 98.Tardy*	0 21 DestOthr	0 56h.OtherPhys
0 103.Sad	0 56f.Stomach	2 45.Nervous	1 35.Worth- less*	0 85.Strange Ideas	2 17.DaDream	0 101.Truant	1 23.DisbSchl	0 58.PickSkin
0 111.With- drawn	0 56g.Vomit	0 47.Conforms*	0 36.GetHurt*	2 TOTAL	2 22.Direct*	0 105.Alcohol Drugs	2 24.Disturbs*	0 59.SleepClass
5 TOTAL	0 TOTAL	0 50.Fearful	1 38.Teased	65 T SCORE	2 41.Impulsv	4 TOTAL	1 27.Jealous	2 73.Irresponsb
63 T SCORE	50 T SCORE	0 52.Guilty	1 48.NotLiked	50 CLIN T	2 45.Nervous	63 T SCORE	1 37.Fights	0 79.SpeechProb
52 CLIN T	44 CLIN T	1 71.SelfConsc	2 62.Clumsy		2 49.Learng*	52 CLIN T	2 53.TalksOut*	1 83.StoresUp
		1 81.HurtCrit*	0 64.Prefers65		1 60.Apathy*		0 57.Attacks	0 91.TalkSuicid
		0 89.Suspic	9 TOTAL		1 61 Poor School		2 67.Disrupts*	0 96.SexPreocc
		0 103.Sad	69 T SCORE		2 62.Clumsy		1 68.Screams	1 99.TooNeat
		0 106.AxPleas*	55 CLIN T		0 72.Messy*		2 74.ShowOff	0 107.DislkSchl
		0 108.Mistake*			2 78.Inatten*		1 76.Explosive*	0 109.Whining
		1 112.Worries			2 80.Stares		2 77.Demanding*	0 110.Unclean
		7 TOTAL			2 92.UnderAch*		2 86.Stubborn	- 113.OtherProb
		61 T SCORE			2 100.Tasks*		2 87.MoodChng	
		49 CLIN T			35 TOTAL		2 93.TalkMuch	
					86 T SCORE		1 94.Teases	
					66 CLIN T		1 95.Temper	
							1 97.Threaten	
							2 104.Loud	
							34 TOTAL	
							77 T SCORE	
							61 CLIN T	

*Items not on Cross-Informant Construct

Profile Type:	WTHDR	SOMAT	SOCIAL	DEL-AGG	With-Thot	Att
ICC:	-.298	-.852	.202	.477**	-.090	.229

** significant ICC with profile type

Figure 5.2. (Continued)

In addition to her ratings on the TRF, Lonnie's teacher completed the Conners Teacher Rating Scale (CTRS; Conners, 1990), which has scales designated as Conduct Problems, Hyperactivity, and Inattentive-Passive, as well as a Hyperactivity Index. The CTRS produced scores in the clinical range for Conduct Problems, Hyperactivity, and the Hyperactivity Index.

In an interview with the school psychologist, Lonnie's teacher reported that he had great difficulty working independently, was disorganized, and failed to complete his daily assignments. She said he often seemed to be "in outer space." When she gave Lonnie instructions, he didn't listen and was easily distracted by other activity in the room. It was difficult to get his attention once he was distracted. The teacher frequently reminded Lonnie to keep working and reprimanded him for inappropriate behavior, ultimately sending him to the principal's office when he became too disruptive. She had tried giving Lonnie stickers or "happy faces" for good days, but this had done little to improve his behavior. Although Lonnie's teacher thought he was a bright boy, she could not understand why he still had trouble with schoolwork after repeating first grade.

Direct Assessment of Lonnie

As suggested in Chapter 2, a teacher's aide used the DOF to rate Lonnie's behavior in the classroom on three occasions. The aide also rated the behavior of two control boys for comparison to Lonnie. On the DOF, Lonnie scored in the clinical range for total problems and the Hyperactive scale, shown earlier in Figure 2.6, but in the normal range for the other five DOF syndromes. The two control boys scored in the normal range on all DOF scales. Lonnie was on-task only 50% of the time, compared to 95% for the two control boys, averaged over the three observation sessions.

By administering the SCICA, the school psychologist could observe Lonnie's behavior and hear Lonnie's own views of his problems and competencies. Lonnie was immediately friendly and talkative. His sense of humor was contagious, as he told jokes, made faces, and gave lengthy descriptions of his exploits in the neighborhood. Despite his gregarious nature, Lonnie reported problems getting along with other children and family members. He admitted fighting with certain children at school, who hit and punched him and called him names. He also said that he was picked on at home by his older sister, who always wanted her own way and bossed him around. Lonnie believed that the fights and arguments were usually started by other children. He could not think of anything he did to provoke the conflicts. Nor could he think of anything he could do to cope with such problems, except to tell his teacher or his mother or to get mad and hit back. "I tattle a lot," Lonnie said. When asked about his wishes, Lonnie said he wanted every Lego set and every kid to be his friend.

Lonnie hated school and wished he could stay home and play every day. He thought most of his schoolwork was boring. He said he always had piles of papers to do and often had to stay in at recess to finish them. Sometimes the teacher sent papers home to complete. Lonnie said his teacher yelled at him a lot for moving around and talking too much. He said it was hard for him to sit still in his seat. However, being one of the "bad kids" at school was good, Lonnie said, because he got happy faces when he behaved and did his work. The only school subject Lonnie liked was art because it was fun. Lonnie also enjoyed puzzles, Lego and other construction toys, and doing craft projects at home.

As the interview progressed, Lonnie became less cooperative and needed encouragement to continue talking and performing the required tasks. Although he said he loved to draw, he resisted drawing his family. Eventually, he drew a picture of his house with himself, mother, and sister each looking out a window. This way, Lonnie said, he only had to draw circles for their heads. While discussing his family drawing, Lonnie acknowledged arguing with his mother and sister, protesting that the rules at home were unfair. Lonnie reported that he was sometimes spanked, but he said he received no other punishments at home. Lonnie said very little about his father except that he visited him on weekends.

Lonnie's behavior changed markedly when he was given standardized achievement tests toward the end of the SCICA. He became very restless, distractible, and unsure of himself. He needed frequent repetitions of directions and questions. On the math test, he often made wrong guesses but then corrected his mistakes on a second try. On the reading recognition test, he carefully sounded out easy words but was reluctant to try more difficult ones. Lonnie wrote only his first name and three simple words for a requested writing sample.

On the SCICA profile, shown in Figure 5.3 (pp. 120-121), Lonnie's scores for total observed problems, total self-reports, Internalizing, and Externalizing were all typical of clinically referred children, with T scores ranging from 50 to 57. Lonnie showed marked peaks on the Anxious and Aggressive Behavior syndromes, with T scores of 66 and 61, respectively,

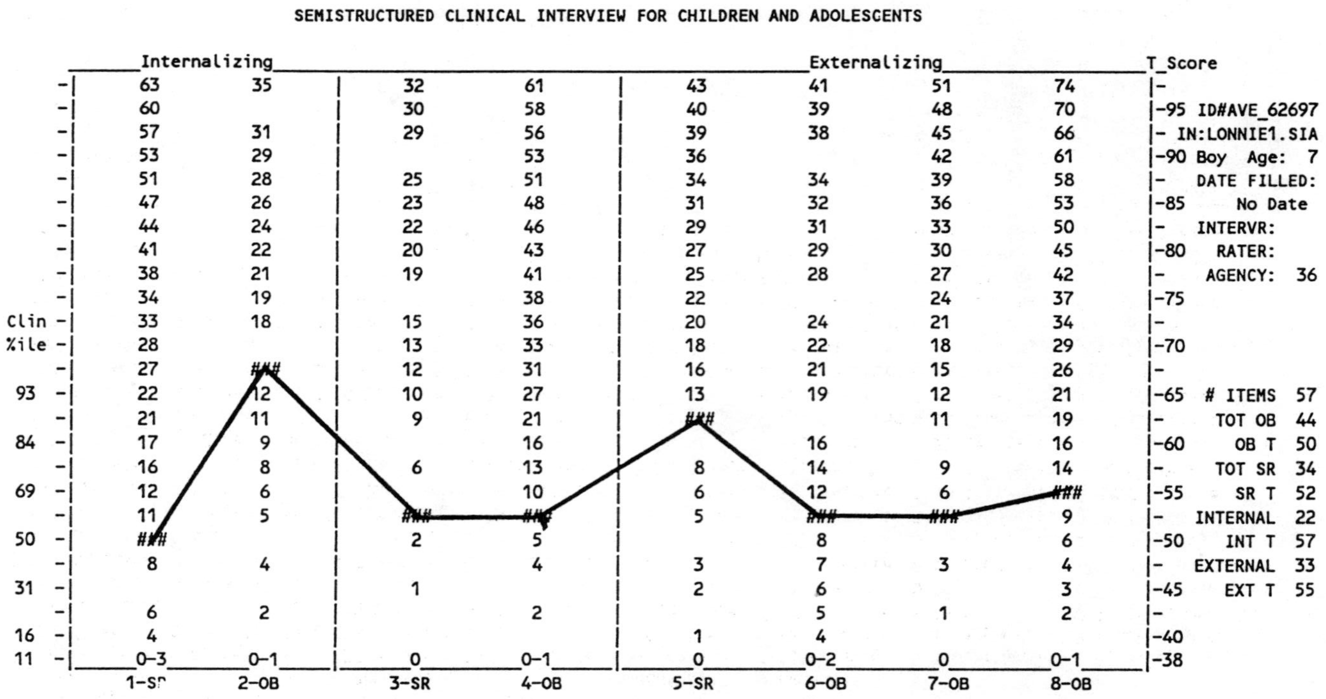

SEMISTRUCTURED CLINICAL INTERVIEW FOR CHILDREN AND ADOLESCENTS

Internalizing

Externalizing

clin %ile									T_Score
	63	35	32	61	43	41	51	74	-95 ID#AVE_62697
	60		30	58	40	39	48	70	- IN:LONNIE1.SIA
	57	31	29	56	39	38	45	66	-90 Boy Age: 7
	53	29		53	36		42	61	- DATE FILLED:
	51	28	25	51	34	34	39	58	-85 No Date
	47	26	23	48	31	32	36	53	- INTERVR:
	44	24	22	46	29	31	33	50	-80 RATER:
	41	22	20	43	27	29	30	45	-
	38	21	19	41	25	28	27	42	- AGENCY: 36
	34	19		38	22		24	37	-75
clin	33	18	15	36	20	24	21	34	-70
%ile	28		13	33	18	22	18	29	-
	27		12	31	16	21	15	26	-
93	22	12	10	27	13	19	12	21	-65 # ITEMS 57
	21	11	9	21			11	19	- TOT OB 44
84	17	9		16		16		16	-60 OB T 50
	16	8	6	13	8	14	9	14	- TOT SR 34
69	12	6		10	6	12	6		-55 SR T 52
	11	5			5			9	- INTERNAL 22
				5		8		6	-50 INT T 57
50	8	4	2	4	3	7	3	4	- EXTERNAL 33
	6	2	1		2	6		3	-45 EXT T 55
31	4			2		5	1	2	-
16					1	4			-40
11	0-3	0-1	0	0-1	0	0-2	0	0-1	-38
	1-SR	2-OB	3-SR	4-OB	5-SR	6-OB	7-OB	8-OB	

Figure 5.3. SCICA profile for Lonnie at age 7.

ANXIOUS/DEPRESSED	ANXIOUS	FAMILY PROBLEMS	WITHDRAWN	AGGRESSIVE BEHAVIOR	ATTENTION PROBLEMS	STRANGE	RESISTANT
0 128.Confused	1 23.Confused	0 135.HarmdPar	0 5.Apathetic	0 122.Mean	1 4.ActYoung	0 1.OverConfid	1 6.Argues
0 134.Lonely	2 29.Difficlt Directns	0 136.Punished	0 9.AvoidsEye	2 130.DisobHom	0 22.Concrete	1 3.Giggles	2 7.AskFeedback
0 137.SelfConsc	1 44.Difficlt Home	1 142.Unfair Home	0 56.NoConver	1 131.DisobSch	1 24.Reverses	1 15.Brags	0 10.Irresponsible
0 141.Fearful	Express	0 143.Unfair School	0 57.NoFantsy	0 132.Impulsiv	1 31.Doesnt Concentr	0 16.BurpFart	0 14.BlameInterv
0 144.Concentr	School	1 151.TooNeat	1 63.NeedCoax	0 140.Suspics	2 32.Doesnt SitStill	0 17.MindOff	2 21.ComplainHard
0 146.Underact	0 46.Doesnt Remember	0 177.HatesPar	0 72.WontTalk	2 145.SitStill	1 33.Distract	0 18.ChewsClth	0 27.Defiant
0 147.Sad	2 50.Fears	0 181.NoAttent	1 73.WTFeelingO	0 155.Destroys OwnThngs	1 38.Fidgets	0 26.Daydreams	0 28.DemandsMet
0 157.Directns	2 52.Confidnc	1 186.NotGet AlongPar	0 74.WontGues	0 156.Destroys Others	0 42.Clumsy	0 30.Disjoint Conversat	0 36.Explosive
1 158.Learning	0 65.Nervous	0 196.Screams	0 77.DontKnow	2 173.Fights	1 45.Understnd	0 35.Exaggerat	0 40.OffTask
0 160.FrMistake	1 68.AnxPleas	0 229.Headache	0 79.Secretiv	0 175.BadComp	0 53.Lapses	1 41.LongRespns	1 43.Guesses
0 162.Fears	1 83.SelfCons	0 234.Stomache	2 80.Overtird	0 178.HateTchr	2 64.NdRepeat	0 51.Jokes	2 48.Impatient
1 164.Guilty	2 102.TooNeat	3 TOTAL	0 82.NoHumor	1 182.NoGuilt	0 66.Twitches	0 55.Leave Toilet	1 49.Impulsive
1 168.OutToGet	0 103.Fearful	54 CLIN T	0 85.Shy	1 188.Attacks	0 67.OutOfSeat	0 71.PlaySexPrt	0 59.OddNoises
0 169.Overtired	0 104.Tremors		1 86.SlowVerb	0 205.Temper	0 88.SpeechPrb	0 75.RepeatActs	0 60.MessyWork
0 171.Worthless	13 TOTAL		1 87.SlowWarm	0 207.Threaten	9 TOTAL	0 91.Strange Behavior	1 61.Misbehaves
3 174.Teased	66 CLIN T		0 89.Stares	9 TOTAL	51 CLIN T	0 92.Strange Ideas	0 76.Resistant
0 179.Nightmare			0 93.Stubborn	61 CLIN T		0 98.Swears	0 78.Screams
1 185.Notliked			0 106.Underact			1 100.TalkMuch	0 84.ShowsOff
1 192.NGetAlong			0 107.Sad			4 TOTAL	0 95.MoodChange
1 193.NoFriends			0 111.Quiet			51 CLIN T	0 97.Suspicious
1 194.SchoolWork			0 114.Withdrawn				0 99.TalksSelf
0 214.Worries			6 TOTAL				0 101.TemperAngry
9 TOTAL			51 CLIN T				0 105.Manipulates
50 CLIN T							0 110.Loud
							1 112.Quits
							0 115.Careless
							11 TOTAL
							55 CLIN T

Figure 5.3. (Continued)

which were above the 84th percentile of the SCICA clinical sample. Lonnie's *T* scores for the remaining six SCICA syndromes, including Attention Problems, ranged from 50 to 55, which were near the 50th percentile for clinically referred children. All SCICA scores were more than one standard deviation above the mean scores obtained by a nonreferred sample (McConaughy & Achenbach, 1994b).

Cognitive Assessment

On the Wechsler Intelligence Scale for Children (WISC-III), Lonnie scored in the high average range for both verbal and performance ability, obtaining a full-scale IQ score of 114. He showed above average ability on subtests of factual information, vocabulary knowledge, and verbal reasoning. These scores were consistent with the school psychologist's observations of good conversational skills during the SCICA, as well as the teacher's impression that Lonnie was a bright boy. Lonnie also scored above average on subtests of visual-spatial skills, perhaps accounting for his interests in construction toys and puzzles. On subtests composing the Freedom From Distractibility Index (Wechsler, 1991), however, Lonnie obtained low average scores. The Gordon Diagnostic System (GDS; Gordon, 1988), which consists of continuous performance tasks administered by a computer, also indicated a shorter attention span and higher impulsivity than normative samples of peers displayed. Despite some scatter on the WISC-III subtests, standardized achievement tests yielded average scores in all areas.

During the WISC-III, the school psychologist noted that Lonnie needed frequent coaxing and praise to continue attempting difficult items. Lonnie also argued about the task requirements and often tried to do things his own way. He showed reasonably good concentration when working with pictures and manipulative materials on nonverbal tasks but was quite restless and distractible during verbal tasks. Allowing Lonnie to take brief walks around the room helped to reduce his restlessness during testing. Awarding stickers for good effort after each WISC-III subtest also improved his cooperation dramatically. Lonnie carefully counted his stickers as they accumulated and showed obvious pride in his accomplishments at the end of the testing session.

Physical Assessment

A recent pediatric exam indicated normal physical development. Medical records revealed normal developmental milestones but a history of ear infections requiring antibiotics until about age 6. The pediatrician had also treated Lonnie for two injuries requiring stitches after bike accidents.

Case Formulation for Lonnie

Lonnie illustrates the value of multiaxial empirically based assessment of attention problems, particularly when parents and teachers express differing opinions about a child's behavior, as did Lonnie's mother and teacher. The CBCL/TRF cross-informant comparisons actually indicated above average parent-teacher agreement on item scores and average parent-teacher agreement on syndrome scores. Lonnie's mother and teacher both endorsed many items on the CBCL/TRF Attention Problems syndromes, producing scores in the clinical range. These results were consistent with scores in the clinical range on the Hyperactivity Index and related scales of the CPRS and CTRS. Classroom observations produced a clinical range score on the DOF Hyperactive syndrome, corroborating the teacher's report. A score at the 50th percentile on the SCICA Attention Problems syndrome also indicated that, even in the one-to-one interaction during the clinical interview, Lonnie manifested attention problems typical of many clinically referred children.

Lonnie's high scores on the empirically based Attention Problems scales, combined with reports from his mother and teacher during interviews, met criteria for a *DSM-IV* diagnosis of ADHD-Combined Type. Although the empirically based procedures were not designed to produce *DSM* diagnoses, their results can support certain diagnoses, as discussed in Chapter 3. For example, on the CBCL, TRF, DOF, and/or SCICA, Lonnie received positive scores on the item, *Can't (doesn't) concentrate, can't (doesn't) pay attention for long,* corresponding to the *DSM-IV* symptom, *often has difficulty sustaining attention in tasks or play activities,* as well as *Can't (doesn't) sit still, restless, or hyperactive* and *Fidgets,* corresponding to the *DSM-IV* symptom, *often fidgets with hands or feet or squirms in seat.* Items scored on one or more of the empirically based measures indicated seven of the nine symptoms listed by *DSM-IV* for inattention and eight of the nine symptoms listed for hyperactivity-impulsivity. These results were consistent with symptoms reported by Lonnie's mother during an interview with the school psychologist.

In addition to current symptoms of inattention and/or hyperactivity-impulsivity, a *DSM-IV* diagnosis of ADHD requires evidence of symptoms before age 7; impairment in two or more settings; and impairment in social, academic, or occupational functioning. Reports from Lonnie's mother and teacher, and his retention in first grade, indicated that at least some symptoms had been apparent since Lonnie entered school. Although Lonnie's mother did not characterize him as hyperactive, she acknowledged that he was always very active and easily distracted. High scores on the CBCL, TRF, CPRS, and CTRS problem scales, combined with low scores on the CBCL School scale and the TRF Adaptive Functioning scale, demonstrated significant impairment in both home and school settings, compared to normative samples of boys his age.

Standardized testing revealed average intelligence and no significant IQ-achievement discrepancies, indicating that Lonnie's reported school problems were not due to low ability or learning disabilities. Nonetheless, Lonnie's high score on the SCICA Anxious syndrome revealed confusion, anxiety, and lack of confidence, which could easily undermine his school performance. Lonnie's negative attitude toward school was especially important to consider in designing educational interventions.

Lonnie also obtained borderline to clinical range scores on the CBCL and TRF Social Problems syndrome, which does not have a direct counterpart in the *DSM*. Both his mother and teacher reported the following problems: *Acts too young for his age, Clings to adults or too dependent, Doesn't get along with other children, Gets teased a lot,* and *Not liked by other children*. During the SCICA, Lonnie gave vivid accounts of his social difficulties and seemed to lack skills for coping with such problems. These findings for Lonnie are consistent with research showing social skills deficits and problems in peer relations among many children with ADHD (Landau & Moore, 1991).

There was less consistency among the different data sources regarding aggressive behavior. Lonnie's mother and teacher both reported that he argued a lot, was disobedient, and sometimes got into fights, but his teacher reported much more aggressive behavior than did his mother. During the SCICA, Lonnie also described fights with other children, which mostly occurred during recess at school. It thus appeared that Lonnie's aggressive behavior was more of a problem at school than at home and was exacerbated by his poor social coping skills revealed during the SCICA.

Interventions for Lonnie

Based on the multiaxial assessment, the school psychologist recommended a combination of pharmacologic treatment and behavioral interventions coordinated between home and school. The preponderance of evidence for the ADHD diagnosis convinced Mrs. Parker that a trial of medication was appropriate. After reading the psychologist's evaluation report, Lonnie's pediatrician began treatment with methylphenidate (Ritalin). The initial scores on the CBCL, TRF, CPRS, and CTRS served as baseline measures of Lonnie's behavior prior to medication. Mrs. Parker and Lonnie's teacher each provided weekly ratings on the CPRS and CTRS, respectively, over an 8-week period. Staff in the pediatrician's office charted scores on the Hyperactivity Index in relation to medication dosages. After 2 weeks, Lonnie's scores on the CPRS and CTRS declined, eventually reaching subclinical levels, except for brief peaks during the Christmas and Easter holidays.

As an additional intervention, Mrs. Parker agreed to participate in a parent training program offered by the mental health providers in her HMO. The program focused on improving parents' strategies for managing oppositional defiant behavior and other problems often associated with ADHD (Barkley, 1987, 1990). Ten weekly sessions were conducted by a mental health counselor for Lonnie's mother and seven other parents.

The school psychologist consulted with Lonnie's teacher to develop classroom accommodations to reduce attention problems and improve Lonnie's organizational skills, as suggested by Abramowitz and O'Leary (1991) and Dawson (1995). Accommodations included (a) breaking academic tasks down into a sequence of small steps; (b) assigning tasks one at a time whenever possible; (c) asking Lonnie to paraphrase directions before beginning a new task; (d) helping Lonnie to verbalize aloud steps and strategies for new or difficult assignments; (e) allowing Lonnie to work in a quiet corner of the classroom for tasks requiring sustained mental effort; and (f) allowing short breaks and physical activity between seat work assignments.

A school-based behavior modification program was implemented to improve Lonnie's on-task behavior and work completion. Following steps recommended by DuPaul and Stoner (1994), a token reinforcement system was tied to menus of daily and weekly rewards. A warning system and time-out procedures were established to reduce disruptive behavior in the classroom. School-home notes were used for weekly communication between Lonnie's mother and teacher, as recommended by Kelley (1990). In addition, the school psychologist enrolled Lonnie in a social skills program (McGinnis & Goldstein, 1984) with several other children in first and second grade. These interventions were maintained for the remaining 7 months of first grade and then reinstated the next year when Lonnie entered second grade.

Outcomes for Lonnie

To assess Lonnie's progress, his mother completed the CBCL/4-18 and his first-grade teacher completed the TRF 6 months (defined as Time 2) after the initial assessment (Time 1). The TRF was also obtained from Lonnie's second-grade teacher 12 months after the initial assessment (Time 3). The Time 2 CBCL/4-18 showed a marked improvement in Lonnie's behavior, with a drop of 20 points in his total problem raw score, bringing it into the normal range. Although Mrs. Parker continued to report some problems on the Social Problems and Attention Problems syndromes at Time 2, scores on both syndromes fell to the normal range.

Figure 5.4 shows Lonnie's scores on the TRF syndromes for the Time 1 assessment (solid line) and subsequent assessments at Time 2 (broken line) and Time 3 (dotted line). On the Time 2 TRF, Lonnie's scores for Attention Problems and Social Problems were in the normal range, owing to decreases in problems previously reported by the same teacher. His score for Aggressive Behavior also decreased slightly but remained in the borderline range. Although it is common for problem scores to decline somewhat over relatively brief periods, the drop in Time 2 CBCL and TRF scores over 6 months demonstrated substantial improvements in problems directly targeted by the medical and educational interventions but less improvement in aggressive behavior.

On the Time 3 TRF obtained from his second-grade teacher, Lonnie's scores were all well within the normal range, indicating even more dramatic improvements in his school behavior. Developmental maturation, changes in the school environment, and interactions with the new teacher may have contributed to the low Time 3 TRF scores, along with beneficial effects of continuing medication and behavioral interventions. Situational changes were especially relevant to the drop in Aggressive Behavior since Lonnie's second-grade teacher reported that one child who had fought with him in first grade had moved out of the school district.

Summary of Lonnie

Lonnie's case illustrates convergence between empirically based assessment of Attention Problems and *DSM-IV* criteria for ADHD in a 7-year-old boy. When he was in first grade, Lonnie obtained clinical range scores on the CBCL and TRF Attention Problems scales, as well as the DOF Hyperactive scale, indicating more problems than are typically reported for boys his age. In addition, observations of Lonnie's behavior during a clinical interview produced a score on the SCICA Attention

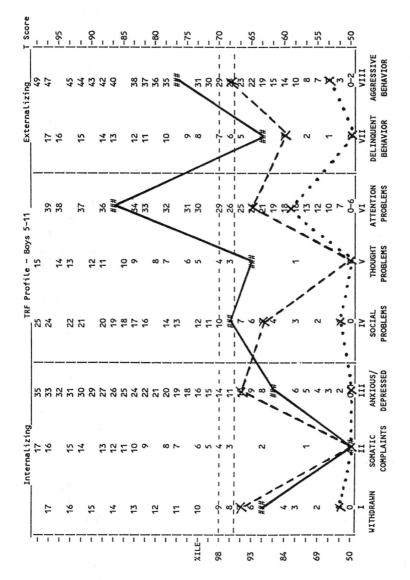

Figure 5.4. Lonnie's TRF problem profile at Time 1 (solid line), Time 2 (broken line), and Time 3 (dotted line).

Problems scale that was at the 50th percentile for clinically referred children. Item scores on the empirically based measures corresponded to seven of the nine symptoms of inattention and eight of the nine symptoms of hyperactivity-impulsivity specified by *DSM-IV* for ADHD. Reports from Lonnie's mother during an interview were consistent with findings from the empirically based measures, as well as providing other necessary information regarding onset, duration, and impairment criteria for ADHD. The *DSM-IV* diagnosis was based on the reported presence of the required symptoms; the CBCL, TRF, and DOF indicated that Lonnie's attention problems were clinically deviant from norms for his age.

The initial assessment of Lonnie led to school interventions and pharmacotherapy for ADHD. However, the empirically based procedures also indicated severe social problems and aggressive behavior in school that were not reflected in the ADHD diagnosis. Identification of these problems led to social skills training and other school interventions that might not have been considered had the focus been restricted to the ADHD diagnosis.

The CBCL and TRF, along with the Conners scales, were later used to assess Lonnie's behavior in response to stimulant medication and to evaluate 6- and 12-month outcomes. Over the 6-month interval, scores on the CBCL and TRF showed substantial improvement in Lonnie's attention and social problems but little change in his aggressive behavior in school. The following year, however, normal range scores on all TRF scales demonstrated marked improvements in Lonnie's behavior in second grade with a new teacher and changes in his peer group. We now turn to the case of 10-year-old Natalie, who manifested a more complex pattern of problems.

CASE 3. NATALIE:
A GIRL WITH ATTENTION AND
SOCIAL PROBLEMS COMBINED
WITH NEGATIVE AFFECTIVITY

Natalie Scott was a frail 10-year-old who was referred to a psychologist for evaluation of her behavioral and emotional functioning. Her fourth-grade teacher was concerned about extreme emotional reactions to minor events in school. The teacher reported that hardly a day went by without Natalie breaking down in tears. Sometimes Natalie cried when assignments seemed too difficult or she didn't understand something. When the teacher gave directions to the whole class, Natalie didn't listen and later needed directions repeated. She was reluctant to try anything on her own and constantly asked for help, even on assignments similar to ones she had done before. At other times, Natalie cried and brooded over conflicts at home or problems getting along with classmates. Making friends was particularly hard for her, because she insisted on their exclusive attention. For example, Natalie would make friends with another girl and then become jealous and hostile whenever her new friend played with someone else. Eventually, each new friend rejected Natalie, leading to complaints to the teacher that no one liked her and no one would play with her.

The school guidance counselor met with Natalie several times to discuss her social problems and invited her to participate in a small peer group on friendship issues. The guidance counselor and teachers also discussed their concerns with Natalie's mother. When these interventions failed to alleviate Natalie's frequent upsets, the school staff recommended an evaluation by a clinical child psychologist who provided contracted services to the school district. The evaluation included cognitive testing, empirically based measures, and interviews with Natalie, her teacher, and Mrs. Scott. Special education staff also administered individualized achievement tests to assess possible learning disabilities.

Parent Reports

Natalie was the third child in an intact middle-class family of five children. Her father worked in the construction business, and her mother worked as a secretary. At the time Natalie was referred for evaluation, her family was experiencing financial difficulties because her father had been laid off due to a slowdown in construction.

CBCL ratings by Mrs. Scott produced a total competence score in the clinical range. Natalie's score on the Activities scale was in the borderline range, whereas her scores on the Social and School scales were at the low end of the normal range. On the Social scale, Mrs. Scott reported that Natalie had only one friend, whom she saw less than once a week. She rated Natalie *worse* for getting along with other children but *about average* for getting along with siblings, behaving with parents, and playing or working alone. These ratings of Natalie's social relationships and her involvement in Girl Scouts and a team sport yielded a score in the low normal range on the Social scale.

Natalie's scores on the CBCL/4-18 problem scales are shown in Figure 5.5 (pp. 130-131). Her total problem and Internalizing scores were in the clinical range, whereas her Externalizing score was in the normal range.

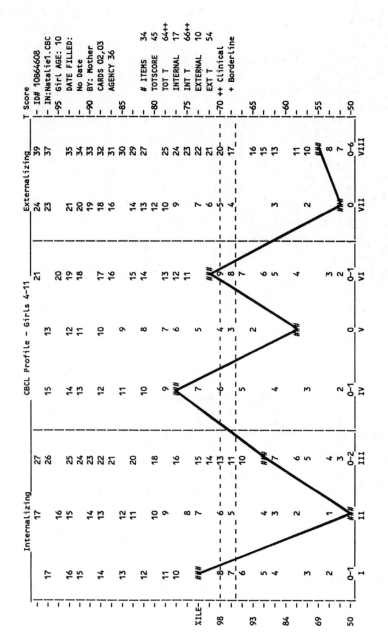

Figure 5.5. CBCL problem profile for Natalie at age 10.

WITHDRAWN	SOMATIC COMPLAINTS	ANXIOUS/ DEPRESSED	SOCIAL PROBLEMS	THOUGHT PROBLEMS	ATTENTION PROBLEMS	DELINQUENT BEHAVIOR	AGGRESSIVE BEHAVIOR	OTHER PROBS
2 42.Rather BeAlone	0 51. Dizzy	2 12.Lonely	2 1. Acts Young	0 9. Mind Off	2 1. Acts Young	0 26.NoGuilt	2 3. Argues	0 5. ActoppSex$
1 65.Won't Talk	0 54. Tired	2 14.Cries	1 11.Clings	0 40.Hears Things	0 8. Concen-trate	0 39.BadCompan	0 7. Brags	0 6. BM Out
2 69.Secret-ive	0 56a.Aches	1 31.FearDoBad	1 25.NotGet Along	0 66.Repeats Acts	2 10.Sit Still	1 43.LieCheat	0 16.Mean	0 15.CruelAnim
	0 56b.Head-aches	0 32.Perfect	1 38.Teased	0 70.Sees Things	0 13.Confuse	0 63.PrefOlder	0 19.DemAttn	0 18.HarmSelf
1 75.Shy	0 56c.Nausea	0 33.Unloved	1 48.Not Liked	0 80.Stares*	2 17.Day-dream	0 67.RunAway	0 20.DestOwn	0 24.NotEat
1 80.Stares	0 56d.Eye	0 34.OutToGet	0 55.Over-Weight*	0 84.Strange Behav	1 41.Impulsv	0 72.SetFires	0 21.DestOthr	0 28.EatNonFood
1 88.Sulks	0 56e.skin	1 35.Worthless	0 62.Clumsy	0 85.Strange Ideas	0 45.Nervous	0 81.StealHome	0 22.DisbHome*	0 29.Fears
0 102.Under-active	0 56f.Stomach	0 45.Nervous	2 64.Prefers Young		2 46.Twitch*	0 82.StealOut	1 23.Disbschl	0 30.FearSchool
0 103.Sad	0 56g.Vomit	0 50.Fearful			0 61.Poor School	0 90.Swears	1 27.Jealous	1 36.Accidents
1 111.With-drawn		1 52.Guilty				1 96.ThnkSex*$	1 37.Fights	0 44.BiteNail
		1 71.Selfconsc			0 45.Nervous	0 101.Truant	0 57.Attacks	0 47.Nightmares
		0 89.Suspic			0 62.Clumsy	0 105.AlcDrugs	1 68.Screams	0 49.Constipate
		1 103.Sad			0 80.Stares	0 106.Vandal*	0 74.ShowOff	0 53.Overeat
		1 112.Worries					0 86.Stubborn	0 56h.OtherPhys
							1 87.MoodChng	0 58.PickSkin
							0 93.TalkMuch	0 59.SexPrtsF$
							0 94.Teases	0 60.SexPrtsM$
							1 95.Temper	0 73.SexProbs$
							0 97.Threaten	0 76.SleepLess
							0 104.Loud	0 77.SleepMore
9 TOTAL	0 TOTAL	8 TOTAL	8 TOTAL	1 TOTAL	10 TOTAL	1 TOTAL	9 TOTAL	0 78.SmearBM
73 T SCORE	50 T SCORE	63 T SCORE	76 T SCORE	58 T SCORE	72 T SCORE	51 T SCORE	55 T SCORE	0 79.SpeechProb
60 CLIN T	40 CLIN T	46 CLIN T	58 CLIN T	44 CLIN T	53 CLIN T	40 CLIN T	40 CLIN T	0 83.StoresUp
								0 91.TalkSuicid
								0 92.SleepWalk
								2 98.ThumbSuck
								0 99.TooNeat
								0 100.SleepProb
								0 107.WetsSelf
								0 108.WetsBed
								0 109.Whining
								0 110.WshOpSex$
								0 113.OtherProb

IX
SEX PROBLEMS
0 TOTAL SCORE
$50 T SCORE
Probs Syndrome

Not in Total Problem Score
*Items not on Cross-Informant Construct   0 2.Allergy   1 4.Asthma

Profile Type:	WTHDR	SOMAT	SOCIAL	DEL-AGG	Delinq
ICC:	.248	-.126	.239	-.435	-.450

No ICCs are significant

Figure 5.5. (Continued)

131

The profile of syndrome scores showed peaks in the clinical range on the Withdrawn, Social Problems, and Attention Problems syndromes. Natalie's scores on the remaining five syndromes were in the normal range, although her score on the Anxious/Depressed syndrome reached the 90th percentile.

In her interview with the psychologist, Mrs. Scott reported that Natalie had developed language and motor skills more slowly than her siblings and still seemed immature for her age. She described Natalie as a quiet, pensive child who was somewhat of a loner. Until age 8, Natalie had been close to her older sister, Jill, and was often included in games with Jill's friends. Both girls attended the same school until Jill advanced to middle school; at that time, Jill expanded her circle of friends and no longer included Natalie in her activities. Natalie then turned her attention to her 6-year-old sister, Karen, or played by herself. She seldom had friends come to her home. When she entered fourth grade, Natalie joined Girl Scouts, but the scout leader reported that she was often tearful and tended to isolate herself from the other girls.

Natalie and her mother often argued about homework assignments and chores. On some days, Natalie would claim that she had no homework or say that she left it at school. On days when Natalie did her homework, she later lost it or forgot to give it to the teacher. Eventually, the teacher sent notes home indicating that Natalie was behind in her schoolwork. Natalie also procrastinated on homework and chores. Her main chores were setting the table and loading the dishwasher. Often Natalie would start one of these chores but then become absorbed in another activity and never finish the original task. Mrs. Scott also felt that Natalie was more easily frustrated than other children in the family, was overly sensitive to criticism, and had a quick temper, all of which added to her difficulties.

When the psychologist queried Mrs. Scott about *DSM-IV* symptoms, she reported several symptoms of Dysthymia, including frequent crying and irritability, low self-esteem, and low energy. These problems had persisted for at least 2 years. In response to questions about ADHD symptoms, Mrs. Scott reported four symptoms of inattention and two symptoms of hyperactivity-impulsivity, but these were too few to qualify for a diagnosis of ADHD.

Teacher Reports

School records indicated that Natalie had repeated first grade and had received remedial reading and math instruction in second grade. By the time she was referred for evaluation, her fourth-grade teacher reported considerable difficulty in math and failure to complete assignments. On the TRF, the teacher rated Natalie's school performance far below grade in math, somewhat below grade in science, but at grade level in other academic areas, producing a total score for academic performance in the clinical range. The teacher's ratings of TRF adaptive functioning also produced a total score in the clinical range. She rated Natalie below typical pupils in terms of how hard she was working, how appropriately she was behaving, how much she was learning, and how happy she was. Figure 5.6 (pp. 134-135) displays Natalie's scores on the TRF problem scales. She scored in the clinical range for total problems and Internalizing and in the borderline clinical range for Externalizing. Natalie's scores on the TRF Anxious/Depressed and Social Problems scales were very high, whereas her scores on the Withdrawn and Attention Problems scales were in the borderline range. Natalie's overall pattern of problems on the TRF fit the Social Problems profile type, as indicated by an ICC of .649.

Direct Assessment of Natalie

During the SCICA administered by the psychologist, Natalie was anxious and tense. She also seemed immature and self-conscious, consistent with reports from her mother and teacher. Natalie often giggled and hesitated in her speech, and she had difficulty concentrating on any one topic or task for long. Her conversation was disjointed and fragmented as she wandered from topic to topic. The psychologist often had to repeat questions or instructions to keep Natalie on-task. Throughout the interview, Natalie squirmed in her seat, fidgeted with her clothes or objects on the table, and occasionally left her seat to handle something across the room.

Natalie was initially reluctant to say anything negative about her experiences at school or home but later discussed her problems more openly. She reported difficulties getting along with other children and making friends, describing one girl as an "off and on" friend, who was a "pain" when she refused to play with Natalie. When this happened, Natalie felt sad and angry but could not think of anything to do to change her friend's behavior. Instead, Natalie tried to befriend a new girl in class. Natalie reported being teased a lot by children at school and by her sisters and brothers at home. She usually tried to ignore the teasing or to avoid children who teased her. Sometimes she tattled to the teachers, but they usually did nothing to intervene. At home, Natalie was teased constantly

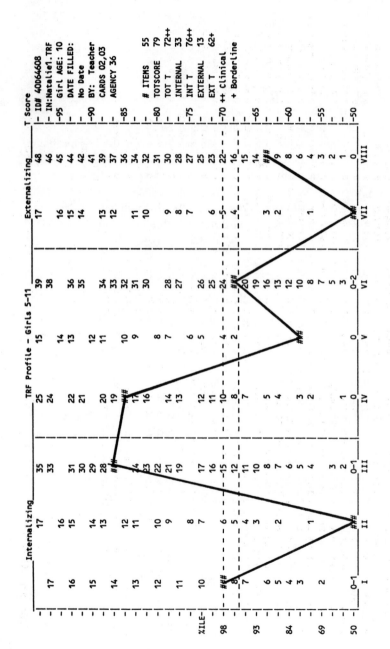

Figure 5.6. TRF problem profile for Natalie at age 10.

134

WITHDRAWN	SOMATIC COMPLAINTS	ANXIOUS/ DEPRESSED	SOCIAL PROBLEMS	THOUGHT PROBLEMS	ATTENTION PROBLEMS	DELINQUENT BEHAVIOR	AGGRESSIVE BEHAVIOR	OTHER PROBS
0 42.Rather BeAlone	0 51.Dizzy	2 12.Lonely	1 1. Acts Young	1 9. Mind Off	1 1. Acts Young	0 26.NoGuilt	1 3. Argues	0 5. ActOppSex
0 65.Won't Talk	0 54. Tired	2 14.Cries	2 11.Clings	0 18.Harms Self*	0 2. Hums*	0 39.Bad Compan	0 6. Defiant*	0 28.EatNonFood
1 69.Secret- ive	0 56a.Aches	1 31.FearDoBad	2 12.Lonely*	0 29.Fears*	2 4. Finish*	0 43.LieCheat	0 7. Brags	0 30.FearSchool
1 75.Shy	0 56b.Head- aches	1 32.Perfect	2 14.Cries*	0 40.Hears Things	1 8.Concentr	0 63.Prefers Older	0 16.Mean	1 44.BiteNail
0 80.Stares	0 56c.Nausea	1 33.Unloved	2 25.NotGet Along	0 66.Repeats Acts	0 10.SitStil	0 82.Steals	2 19.DemAttn	0 46.Twitch
2 88.Sulks	0 56d.Eye	1 34.OutToGet	1 33.Unlove*	0 70.Sees Things	1 13.Confuse	0 90.Swears	0 20.DestOwn	0 55.Overweight
1 102.Under- active	0 56e.Skin	2 35.Worthless	1 34.OutTo Get*	– 84.Strange Behav	2 15.Fidget*	0 98.Tardy*	0 21.DestOthr	0 56h.OtherPhys
	0 56f.Stomach	2 45.Nervous	2 35.Worth- less*	– 85.Strange Ideas	1 17.DaDream	0 101.Truant	0 23.DisbSchl	0 58.PickSkin
	0 56g.Vomit	0 47.Conforms*	1 36.HurtCrit*		2 22.Direct*	0 105.Alcohol Drugs	0 24.Disturbs*	0 59.SleepClass
		0 50.Fearful	2 38.Teased		0 41.Impulsv		2 27.Jealous	2 73.Irresponsb
		1 52.Guilty	1 48.NotLiked		2 45.Nervous		1 37.Fights	0 79.SpeechProb
		2 71.SelfConsc	1 62.Clumsy		1 49.Learng*		0 53.TalksOut*	0 83.StoresUp
		2 81.HurtCrit*	1 64.Prefers59		1 60.Apath*		0 57.Attacks	1 91.TalkSuicid
		0 89.Suspic			1 61.Poor school		0 67.Disrupts*	0 96.SexPreocc
		2 103.Sad			1 62.Clumsy		0 68.Screams	0 99.TooNeat
		1 106.AxPleas*			1 72.Messy*		0 74.ShowOff	1 107.DisLkSchl
		2 108.Mistake*			1 78.Inatten*		1 76.Explosive*	1 109.Whining
		1 112.Worries			0 80.Stares		2 77.Demanding*	0 110.Unclean
					1 92.UnderAch*		2 86.Stubborn	0 113.OtherProb
					2 100.Tasks*		1 87.MoodChng	
							0 93.TalkMuch	
							0 94.Teases	
							1 95.Temper	
							0 97.Threaten	
							0 104.Loud	
9 TOTAL	0 TOTAL	26 TOTAL	18 TOTAL	1 TOTAL	21 TOTAL	0 TOTAL	13 TOTAL	
70 T SCORE	50 T SCORE	86 T SCORE	85 T SCORE	59 T SCORE	67 T SCORE	50 T SCORE	64 T SCORE	
60 CLIN T	43 CLIN T	77 CLIN T	73 CLIN T	47 CLIN T	52 CLIN T	40 CLIN T	48 CLIN T	

*Items not on Cross-Informant Construct

Profile Type:	WTHDR	SOMAT	SOCIAL	DEL-AGG	With-Thot	Att
ICC:	.174	.124	.649**	–.314	.280	–.248

** Significant ICC with profile type

Figure 5.6. (Continued)

by her siblings, which often led to fights and scolding by their parents. Eventually, all the children would be sent to their rooms. Natalie admitted crying a lot in school, mostly because she thought the work was too hard. Other children teased her when she cried. She described math as her hardest subject, especially multiplication and division, which she didn't understand. Natalie often had to stay in for recess or after school to finish her work, but she liked getting help from the teacher. At home, however, Natalie's parents yelled at her about school work and did little to help her. Instead of working, Natalie wished kids could have pizza parties in school and do art all day. During achievement tests administered at the end of the SCICA, Natalie became extremely restless, had difficulty concentrating, and often guessed on math problems.

As shown in Figure 5.7 (pp. 138-139), Natalie's SCICA profile yielded scores above the 70th percentile for clinically referred children on four syndromes. Her high score on the Anxious/Depressed syndrome reflected self-reported social and learning problems, including getting teased, not getting along with other children, having no friends, poor school work, and worries. On the Anxious, Attention Problems, and Strange syndromes, her high scores reflected the psychologist's observations of her behavior during the interview. In contrast, her low score on the Withdrawn syndrome reflected her willingness to talk about her problems with an understanding and supportive adult. Natalie's T scores of 48 to 57 for total observations, total self-reports, Internalizing, and Externalizing were similar to the mean scores of the SCICA clinical sample.

Cognitive Assessment

On the WISC-III, Natalie scored in the average range for both verbal and performance ability, obtaining a full scale IQ score of 96. She showed average to above average ability on all WISC-III subtests, except the three that made up the Freedom from Distractibility Index (Wechsler, 1991). Below average scores for numerical concentration, auditory attention span, and fine motor speed (Coding) were consistent with attention problems observed during the SCICA and reported by Natalie's mother and teacher. Achievement testing also produced below average scores in mathematics, but average scores in other academic skills.

Physical Assessment

Medical records indicated developmental delays in language and motor skills. Natalie also had a history of ear infections and fluid build-up that necessitated periodic antibiotics, plus tympanic membrane tube placements until age 5. At age 10, tests of hearing were within normal limits. Natalie wore glasses for reading and distance vision. A recent pediatric exam indicated normal physical health.

Case Formulation for Natalie

Like Lonnie's in the previous case illustration, Natalie's CBCL and TRF produced borderline to clinical range scores on the Attention Problems and Social Problems syndromes. Cross-informant comparisons showed good agreement between parent and teacher reports, as indicated by above-average *Q* correlations for item and syndrome scores.

Unlike Lonnie, however, Natalie failed to meet criteria for a *DSM-IV* diagnosis of ADHD. The interview with Mrs. Scott, plus the CBCL, TRF, and SCICA, indicated five *DSM-IV* symptoms of inattention and five symptoms of hyperactivity-impulsivity, which failed to meet diagnostic criteria. Yet, scores at or above the 95th percentile on the CBCL and TRF Attention Problems syndromes indicated deviance compared to normative samples of girls.

Natalie also obtained a score above the 70th percentile for clinically referred children on the SCICA Attention Problems scale, as well as below-average scores on the WISC-III distractibility factor. The results of the empirically based measures and cognitive testing thus illustrate the disadvantages of applying the *DSM*'s uniform diagnostic criteria to both genders. As indicated by research reviewed in Chapter 3, lower cutpoints may be needed for diagnoses of ADHD in girls, because uniform cutpoints for both genders require that girls be more deviant from normative samples of peers than boys need to be. Similar problems have been found in applying uniform cutpoints to boys and girls for *DSM* diagnoses of CD (Zoccolillo, 1993).

Although Natalie did not meet diagnostic criteria for ADHD, she did meet criteria for a *DSM-IV* diagnosis of Dysthymia. In the interview with the psychologist, Natalie's mother reported persistent depressed mood and irritability, plus low self-esteem and low energy. On the empirically based Anxious/Depressed syndrome, Natalie scored in the clinical range on the TRF and at the 90th percentile on the CBCL. She also scored above the 70th percentile on the SCICA Anxious/Depressed scale, compared to a clinical sample. Natalie's mother and teacher agreed in reporting problems such as complaining of loneliness, crying a lot, fears of doing something bad, feeling worthless, feeling guilty, and being self-conscious.

138

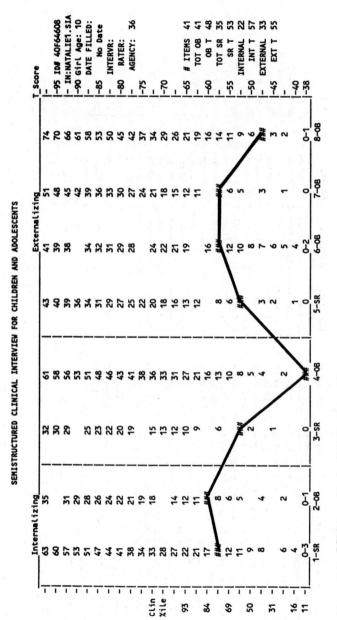

Figure 5.7. SCICA profile for Natalie at age 10.

Profile scoring form (rotated). Each column lists a syndrome scale with item scores.

ANXIOUS/DEPRESSED
- 0 128.Confused
- 0 134.Lonely
- 0 137.SelfConsc
- 0 141.Fearful
- 0 144.Concentr
- 0 146.Underact
- 0 147.Sad
- 0 157.Directns
- 2 158.Learning
- 0 160.FrMistake
- 3 162.Fears
- 0 164.Guilty
- 0 168.OutToGet
- 0 169.Overtired
- 0 171.Worthless
- 3 174.Teased
- 0 179.Nightmare
- 0 185.NotLiked
- 2 192.NgetAlong
- 3 193.NoFriends
- 1 194.SchoolWork
- 1 214.Worries
- 13 TOTAL
- 56 CLIN T

ANXIOUS
- 0 23.Confused
- 0 29.Difficlt Directns
- 0 44.Difficlt Express
- 0 46.Doesnt Remember
- 1 50.Fears
- 0 52.Confidnc Mistakes Learning
- 3 65.Nervous
- 1 68.AnxPleas
- 2 83.SelfCons
- 0 102.TooNeat
- 3 103.Fearful
- 3 104.Tremors
- 9 TOTAL
- 60 CLIN T

FAMILY PROBLEMS
- 0 135.HarmdPar
- 0 136.Punished
- 2 142.Unfair Home
- 0 143.Unfair School
- 0 151.TooNeat
- 0 177.HatesPar
- 0 181.NoAttent
- 1 186.NotGet AlongPar
- 0 196.Screams
- 0 229.Headache
- 0 234.Stomache
- 3 TOTAL
- 54 CLIN T

WITHDRAWN
- 0 5.Apathetic
- 0 9.AvoidsEye
- 0 56.NoConver
- 0 57.NoFantsy
- 0 63.NeedCoax
- 0 72.WontTalk
- 0 73.WTFeeling
- 0 74.WontGues
- 0 77.DontKnow
- 0 79.Secretiv
- 0 80.Overtird
- 0 82.NoHumor
- 0 85.Shy
- 0 86.SlowVerb
- 0 87.SlowWarm
- 0 89.Stares
- 0 93.Stubborn
- 0 106.Underact
- 0 107.Sad
- 0 111.Quiet
- 0 114.Withdrawn
- 0 TOTAL
- 38 CLIN T

AGGRESSIVE BEHAVIOR
- 2 122.Mean
- 2 130.Disobhom
- 1 131.DisobSch
- 3 132.Impulsiv
- 0 140.Suspics
- 3 145.SitStill
- 0 155.Destroys OwnThngs
- 0 156.Destroys Others
- 0 173.Fights
- 0 175.BadComp
- 0 178.HateTchr
- 0 182.NoGuilt
- 2 188.Attacks
- 2 205.Temper
- 0 207.Threaten
- 5 TOTAL
- 53 CLIN T

ATTENTION PROBLEMS
- 2 4.ActYoung
- 0 22.Concrete
- 1 24.Reverses
- 3 31.Doesnt Concentr
- 2 32.Doesnt SitStill
- 0 33.Distract
- 2 38.Fidgets
- 0 42.Clumsy
- 0 45.Understnd
- 0 53.Lapses
- 0 64.NdRepeat
- 0 66.Twitches
- 2 67.OutOfSeat
- 0 88.SpeechPrb
- 14 TOTAL
- 58 CLIN T

STRANGE
- 0 1.OverConfid
- 2 3.Giggles
- 0 15.Brags
- 0 16.BurpFart
- 0 17.MindOff
- 0 18.ChewsClth
- 0 26.Daydreams
- 3 30.Disjoint Conversat
- 0 35.Exaggerat
- 1 41.LongRespns
- 1 51.Jokes
- 0 55.Leave Toilet
- 2 71.PlaySexPrt
- 0 75.RepeatActs
- 0 91.Strange Behavior
- 0 92.Strange Ideas
- 0 98.Swears
- 3 100.TalkMuch
- 9 TOTAL
- 59 CLIN T

RESISTANT
- 0 6.Argues
- 1 7.AskFeedback
- 0 10.Irresponsible
- 0 14.BlameInterv
- 0 21.ComplainHard
- 0 27.Defiant
- 1 28.DemandsMet
- 0 36.Explosive
- 1 40.OffTask
- 0 43.Guesses
- 0 48.Impatient
- 1 49.Impulsive
- 0 59.OddNoises
- 0 60.MessyWork
- 0 61.Misbehaves
- 0 76.Resistant
- 0 78.Screams
- 0 84.ShowsOff
- 0 95.MoodChange
- 0 97.Suspicious
- 1 99.TalksSelf
- 0 101.TemperAngry
- 0 105.Manipulates
- 0 110.Loud
- 0 112.Quits
- 0 115.Careless
- 5 TOTAL
- 49 CLIN T

Figure 5.7. (Continued)

139

Her teacher reported several additional problems, including unhappiness, fearfulness, and worries.

The SCICA further revealed Natalie's intense feelings of being victimized by teasing from peers and siblings and her helplessness in preventing teasing. She also described intense, jealous attachments to other girls, which eventually alienated most new friends. Natalie's poor coping skills and unsuccessful attempts to form lasting friendships helped to account for deviant scores on the CBCL and TRF Withdrawn and Social Problems syndromes. Although these syndromes have no direct counterparts in the *DSM,* they reflect problems that were important to consider in planning interventions, along with the attention problems indicated by the CBCL and TRF and emotional distress reflected in the diagnosis of Dysthymia.

Interventions for Natalie

As with Lonnie, the multiaxial assessment of Natalie provided a basis for multifaceted interventions. High scores on the CBCL and TRF Withdrawn and Social Problems syndromes provided evidence of the SED characteristic of *inability to build or maintain satisfactory interpersonal relationships with peers and teachers.* High scores on the TRF and SCICA Anxious/Depressed syndromes, plus the diagnosis of Dysthymia, provided evidence of the SED characteristic of *a general pervasive mood of unhappiness or depression.* The deviance of Natalie's CBCL and TRF scores from those of her peers showed that she met the SED severity criteria, while parent and teacher reports indicated that her problems had existed for a long period of time and had adverse effects on her educational performance. Low scores on standardized math achievement tests and low productivity in class provided further evidence of adverse effects. Because previous school interventions had produced little change in Natalie's behavior and school performance, the MDT concluded that she was in need of special education services.

Given the SED determination, an Individualized Education Program (IEP) was designed for Natalie that included special instruction in math, combined with behavioral interventions and classroom accommodations. A behavioral incentive plan was developed to improve her effort and on-task behavior. Following Goldstein's (1995) recommendations, a contingency contract was established, specifying target behaviors and a menu of reinforcers identified jointly by Natalie, her teacher, and the psychologist. Potential rewards included special activities and adult attention, as well as material rewards. Natalie's assignments in math were also modified to reduce her workload. School-home notes (Kelley, 1990) provided daily communications with her parents regarding homework assignments and positive comments on her school performance. To improve her coping strategies and peer relations, Natalie was enrolled in a social skills training program (McGinnis & Goldstein, 1984) conducted by the school guidance counselor. The guidance counselor also met with Natalie on an ad hoc basis to help her solve conflicts with peers. To address family issues, Natalie and her parents were referred to a counselor in a community mental health center. The counselor worked on improving self-esteem in individual sessions and met with the family to negotiate strategies for reducing teasing and fighting among the siblings.

Outcomes for Natalie

When Natalie was 13 years old (designated as Time 2), the school MDT obtained a 3-year reevaluation, as required by the IDEA and state special education regulations. The evaluation included the CBCL from Mrs. Scott, TRFs from Natalie's seventh-grade math and home economics teachers, and the YSR. Individual achievement tests were also administered to assess her academic progress. During the 3-year interval between Times 1 and 2, Natalie had an IEP focusing on math instruction, social skills training, behavioral interventions, and classroom accommodations. Natalie and her family also met with a mental health counselor for six sessions but then dropped out of treatment.

Natalie's scores on several CBCL problem scales declined from age 10 (Figure 5.5) to age 13, although her profile pattern remained similar at both ages. Her scores on the Withdrawn syndrome, Internalizing, and total problems declined to the normal range, but her scores on the Social Problems and Attention Problems syndromes were in the borderline range. Her score on the Anxious/Depressed syndrome was in the normal range, as it was at Time 1, although Mrs. Scott reported that Natalie still complained of loneliness, cried, worried, and was nervous and self-conscious.

Figure 5.8 shows the Time 2 TRFs obtained from Natalie's math teacher (solid line) and home economics teacher (broken line). Her scores on the Anxious/Depressed and Social Problems syndromes dropped markedly from the Time 1 TRF (Figure 5.6), even though they remained in the borderline to clinical range on both TRFs. Scores on the Withdrawn and Attention Problems syndromes dropped from the borderline range at Time 1 to the normal range at Time 2. On the Time 2 Attention Problems

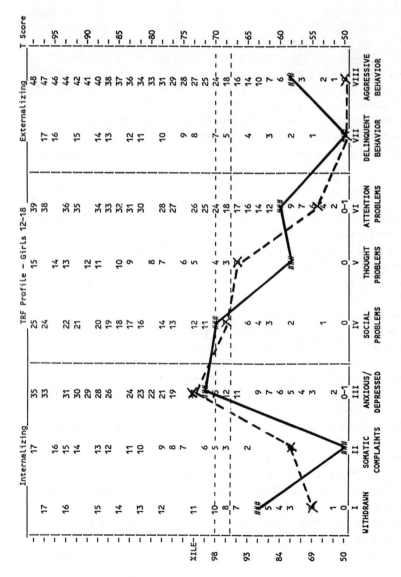

Figure 5.8. TRF profiles for Natalie at age 13. Math teacher (solid line); home economics teacher (broken line).

142

syndrome, however, both teachers rated Natalie as acting young, having difficulty concentrating, fidgeting, and nervous. The math teacher reported additional problems, including failing to finish things, being confused, difficulty following directions, difficulty learning, poor school work, and underachievement, consistent with low average scores on math achievement tests.

In contrast to the Time 2 CBCL and TRFs, Natalie's YSR profile produced normal range scores on all syndromes. This suggested that she viewed her behavior and emotions much more positively than did her mother and teachers. Or perhaps, at age 13, she was less willing to report problems on the YSR than she was during the SCICA at age 10. Nonetheless, Natalie did acknowledge several problems of the Social Problems syndrome, including being too dependent, not getting along with other children, being teased, and preferring younger children. She also scored five of the nine Attention Problems items as *somewhat or sometimes true.*

Summary of Natalie

Natalie's case illustrates a complex pattern of attention and social problems plus negative affectivity in a 10-year-old girl who was reevaluated at age 13. At age 10, Natalie obtained borderline to clinical range scores on the CBCL and TRF Attention Problems and Social Problems scales. She also obtained a score above the 70th percentile on the SCICA Attention Problems scale compared to clinically referred children and low scores on WISC-III subtests measuring distractibility. In spite of the attention problems indicated by the empirically based measures, Natalie failed to meet *DSM-IV* cutpoints for the number of symptoms required for a diagnosis of ADHD. This was in contrast to 7-year-old Lonnie, who met criteria for ADHD, Combined type. Natalie's failure to meet *DSM-IV* criteria for ADHD illustrates the disadvantages of requiring identical diagnostic cutpoints for boys and girls.

Natalie did qualify for a *DSM-IV* diagnosis of Dysthymia, due to her depressed mood, irritability, low self-esteem, and other symptoms reported by her mother. Her clinical range scores on the TRF Anxious/Depressed syndrome from ratings by her teacher and her high score on the SCICA Anxious/Depressed syndrome were consistent with the Dysthymia diagnosis.

The initial assessment of Natalie identified her as a student with SED according to special education criteria. This led to an IEP designed to address her emotional problems in school and to improve her academic performance and social skills. Natalie and her family were also referred to a counselor in a community mental health center. However, they discontinued counseling after six sessions.

The 3-year reevaluation produced a mixed picture of Natalie's behavioral/emotional functioning as she entered adolescence. A dramatic drop in scores on the TRF Anxious/Depressed and Social Problems scales, and some decline on the TRF Withdrawn scale, suggested beneficial effects of the school interventions, particularly social skills training and school-based counseling. Similarly, the drop in the TRF Attention Problems score indicated improvements in Natalie's attention and organizational skills, which her IEP had targeted for improvement via behavioral incentives, classroom accommodations, and individualized assistance in math. As in Lonnie's case, developmental maturation and relationships with new teachers could also have contributed to Natalie's improved functioning in the school setting.

Despite the drop in Time 2 TRF scores on several syndromes, Natalie's scores remained deviant on the TRF Anxious/Depressed and CBCL/TRF Social Problems syndromes. These results indicated persistent negative affectivity and social problems, consistent with longitudinal research demonstrating strong stability for these syndromes. Natalie's deviant score on the CBCL Attention Problems scale at Time 2 is also consistent with longitudinal findings showing strong stability in parent ratings of this syndrome, as well as the greater variety of later problems reported for girls than for boys with attention problems. At age 13, several items scored on the CBCL and TRF Attention Problems scales suggested ADHD symptoms, but the number of symptoms failed to meet cutpoints for a diagnosis. Natalie also endorsed five items on the YSR Attention Problems scale, although her total score on this syndrome was in the normal range. Natalie's persistent negative affectivity and social problems continued to warrant concern and may have overshadowed attention problems, thus illustrating difficulties in choosing among categorical diagnoses for children who exhibit complex patterns of co-occurring problems.

SUMMARY

Two cases were presented to illustrate multiaxial empirically based assessment of elementary school children. Both Lonnie and Natalie manifested attention problems, social problems, and poor school performance, but they differed in important ways that were documented via empirically based assessment.

According to multiple kinds of data, 7-year-old Lonnie manifested more than enough problems of inattention and hyperactivity-impulsivity to qualify for a diagnosis of ADHD Combined Type. In addition, his TRF and SCICA revealed serious aggressive behavior. Reassessments with the empirically based procedures following interventions showed marked improvements in Lonnie's attention problems and social problems over a 6-month period, although his TRF Aggressive Behavior score remained in the borderline clinical range. However, after Lonnie had advanced to a new grade and no longer had contact with a troublesome peer, a 12-month reassessment showed that even his TRF Aggressive Behavior score declined to the normal range.

When initially assessed, 10-year-old Natalie obtained deviant scores on the Withdrawn, Social Problems, and Attention Problems scales scored from both the CBCL/4-18 and TRF. She also obtained a very deviant score on the TRF Anxious/Depressed scale, which was consistent with her high scores on the Anxious/Depressed and Anxious syndromes of the SCICA. The findings clearly supported eligibility for special education services under the SED category, plus a *DSM* diagnosis of Dysthymia, but Natalie's attention problems and social problems did not meet criteria for any *DSM* diagnoses. Following special school services, a 3-year reassessment showed a considerable reduction in problems, although Natalie's profile patterns remained quite similar, and she remained somewhat deviant on the TRF Anxious/Depressed scale, the CBCL Attention Problems scale, and the Social Problems scales of both the TRF and CBCL.

Despite some similarities in problems, Lonnie and Natalie illustrate important differences in overall patterns that were identified at initial and outcome assessments with the empirically based procedures. Furthermore, Natalie's persistently deviant score on the Attention Problems syndrome may reflect the traitlike nature of attention problems in some girls whose behavior fails to meet *DSM* criteria for ADHD.

6

CASE ILLUSTRATIONS FOR ADOLESCENTS

In adolescence, assessment is complicated by the increasing number of informants and by the increasing differentiation of adolescents' own views of their problems from the views of their parents and teachers. Because most adolescents are in departmentalized school programs, reports from multiple teachers can be used to identify consistencies and inconsistencies in school behavior. In addition to interviews and observations, the YSR adds an important component of direct assessment, which may reveal problems and concerns that are not apparent to others. On the other hand, if the YSR indicates fewer problems than are consistently evident in other reports, this suggests that the adolescent may be unaware of problems reported by others or may avoid acknowledging such problems. In either case, interviews with adolescents can then be used to explore their perceptions of their problems and the feasibility of different interventions.

In this chapter, we first return to the case of Kyle, who was introduced at age 12 in Chapters 1 and 2 to illustrate the CBCL, TRF, and SCICA. We summarize Kyle's prior history and assessment at age 12, describe interventions and events between ages 12 and 15, and present results of his reassessment at age 15. After discussing Kyle, we turn to the case of Julie, who was assessed at ages 10, 14, and 15. In addition to illustrating multiaxial assessment of adolescents, the cases of Kyle and Julie portray the developmental course of their competencies and problems.

146

CASE 1. KYLE:
AN ADOLESCENT SHOWING
PERSISTENT AGGRESSIVE BEHAVIOR
(continued from Chapter 2)

Kyle Conner was the oldest child living with his mother and stepfather, Pat and John Conner, and his two younger half-sisters. As indicated in Chapter 1, Kyle's assessment at age 12 began with a visit to the family pediatrician prompted by his sixth-grade teacher's complaints of disruptive behavior in school. Mrs. Conner was also having increasing difficulty dealing with Kyle's behavior and mood swings at home. Low competence and high problem scores on the CBCL from Mrs. Conner led to a referral to the mental health service of the family's HMO for a more comprehensive assessment.

In addition to the CBCL completed by Mrs. Conner, the HMO psychologist obtained a CBCL from Mr. Conner, TRFs from two sixth-grade teachers, and the YSR from Kyle, as well as administering the SCICA to Kyle. Figures 1.1 and 1.2 showed scores on the CBCL competence and problem scales from ratings by Mrs. Conner, and Figure 2.1 showed scores on the TRF problem scales from ratings by Kyle's math teacher. Cross-informant comparisons, shown in Figure 2.3, indicated Aggressive Behavior scores in the clinical range on CBCLs completed by both parents and TRFs from both teachers. Both CBCLs and one TRF also yielded borderline to clinical range scores for Delinquent Behavior, which included scores of 1 or 2 for lacking guilt, hanging around kids who get in trouble, lying or cheating, stealing, swearing, and being tardy to school. The CBCL from Mrs. Conner yielded high scores for the Thought Problems syndrome; one TRF yielded high scores for the Anxious/Depressed and Social Problems syndromes.

Kyle's YSR scores, shown in Figure 2.3, contrasted markedly with his CBCL and TRF scores. His YSR yielded borderline scores on the Externalizing and Withdrawn scales, but normal range scores on all other scales. However, Kyle's behavior ˙and self-reports during the SCICA (Figure 2.5) yielded high scores on the Aggressive Behavior, Anxious/Depressed, and Strange scales compared to other clinically referred children.

As discussed in Chapter 2, the results of the multiaxial assessment of Kyle at age 12 led to a *DSM-IV* diagnosis of CD. The empirically based measures, plus information from the HMO psychologist's interview with Kyle's mother, provided evidence for at least 4 of the 15 behaviors listed for CD: *often bullies, threatens, or intimidates others; often initiates physical fights; often lies to obtain goods or favors or to avoid obligations; and has stolen things of nontrivial value without confronting a victim.* Kyle's high scores on the Aggressive Behavior and Delinquent Behavior syndromes supported the CD diagnosis, consistent with research findings discussed in Chapter 3. Mrs. Conner's reports of fighting, lying, and stealing as early as age 6 indicated that Kyle met criteria for Childhood-Onset CD.

Additional Assessment and Interventions for Kyle at Age 12

At the request of Kyle's parents, the HMO psychologist submitted her report to the school MDT involved in Kyle's case. To further assess Kyle's cognitive and academic functioning, the school psychologist administered the WISC-III and interviewed Kyle's teachers, and the special educator administered achievement tests. Combining information from the HMO psychologist and the school-based assessment, the MDT determined that Kyle's pattern of problems met special education criteria for SED. Low scores on the CBCL Social scale and high scores on the CBCL and TRF Social Problems and YSR Withdrawn scales all provided evidence of the SED characteristic of *an inability to build or maintain satisfactory relationships with peers and teachers.* High scores on the CBCL, TRF, and SCICA Aggressive Behavior, CBCL Thought Problems, and SCICA Strange scales provided evidence of *inappropriate types of behavior or feelings under normal circumstances.* The CD diagnosis was also indicative of inappropriate behavior, although the relevance of CD diagnoses to SED criteria has been hotly debated (e.g., Skiba & Grizzle, 1991, 1992; Slenkovich, 1992). There was also some evidence of *a general pervasive mood of unhappiness,* as indicated by high scores on the TRF and SCICA Anxious/Depressed scales.

Borderline to clinical range scores on the CBCL, TRF, and YSR total problem, Internalizing, Externalizing, and syndrome scales all demonstrated that Kyle displayed problems to a marked degree, compared to normative samples. SCICA clinical T scores greater than one standard deviation above the mean scores obtained by a nonreferred sample also documented the severity of problems revealed during the clinical interview. The histories obtained from Kyle's mother and teachers indicated that his problems had existed for a long period of time.

The WISC-III indicated average to high-average ability and achievement and no specific learning disabilities that might interfere with educational performance. However, there was considerable evidence that Kyle's emotional and behavioral problems produced adverse effects on educational performance in terms of many incomplete assignments, detentions and suspensions, and failing grades in three subjects, plus low scores on the CBCL School and TRF Academic Performance and Adaptive Functioning scales. Kyle's average scores on standardized achievement tests further supported the MDT's conclusion that SED, rather than lack of knowledge, was responsible for his school problems and failing grades. The determination of SED justified an IEP that included behavioral and academic interventions. Following Goldstein's (1995) recommendations, the MDT team designed a behavior modification plan to reduce aggressive and oppositional behavior. The plan included the following components: (a) clearly defined target behaviors; (b) a system for awarding points when behavioral goals were achieved; (c) clearly specified rewards and consequences; (d) a menu of rewards, including both material and social rewards; (e) a clear warning system regarding undesired behavior; (f) time-out procedures; and (g) meetings with a designated adult to develop problem-solving strategies. A room near the school guidance office was designated as a time-out area. After Kyle served time-out, he met with the guidance counselor to discuss the situation and generate alternative strategies for similar situations in the future.

Kyle's low scores on the CBCL total competence and Social scales, plus high scores on the TRF Social Problems scale, indicated a need for social skills training. Kyle was enrolled in a school program with several peers, using skill streaming and *The Prepare Curriculum* developed by Goldstein and colleagues (Goldstein, 1988; McGinnis, Goldstein, Sprafkin, Gershaw, & Klein, 1980). Kyle's parents and teachers also used a notebook to communicate daily about his behavior and academic productivity. Time management procedures and study plans were coordinated between home and school, using materials provided by Kuepper (1987).

Kyle and his family returned to the HMO mental health service for individual and family therapy. Cognitive behavioral therapy was employed (Kendall & Panichelli-Mindel, 1995) to address Kyle's tendency to deny problems, as shown by low scores on the YSR, as well as his paranoid tendencies and quickness to blame others, which were revealed by the SCICA. The HMO psychologist also used parent training techniques developed by Kazdin and colleagues (Kazdin, 1987; Kazdin, Esveldt-Dawson, French, & Unis, 1987) to help Mr. and Mrs. Conner manage Kyle's aggressive and noncompliant behavior at home.

Kyle's Course From Age 12 to 15

Many changes occurred in Kyle's life from age 12 to 15. When he was 13, the family moved to a rural area to accommodate a change in Mr. Conner's employment. This meant a change to a new school and new classmates in seventh grade. The move also produced changes in Kyle's IEP, although he was still classified as a student with SED. Kyle continued to receive individual assistance in study skills and in planning homework, and he remained on a point system for work completion. However, the behavior modification plan and social skills interventions provided in his former school were not continued in his new school.

Mrs. Conner reported that Kyle's behavior improved for a while after the IEP was developed and the family received therapy at the HMO. After the family moved, however, Kyle's associations with a group of older boys led to repeated incidents of staying out late and experimenting with alcohol and drugs. He became more openly defiant, which led to heated conflicts with both parents. When his parents attempted to impose rules, Kyle threatened to run away or talked about suicide, but he never made any suicide attempts.

At age 14, Kyle went to live with his biological father, who had re-established contact in the previous year. However, Kyle's father provided little supervision, and Kyle was involved in two automobile accidents while driving without a license. He also got in trouble with the police for fighting and stealing cigarettes. Six months later, after a beating by his father, Kyle asked to return to the Conners' home.

Reassessment of Kyle at Age 15

When Kyle was 15, the MDT at his high school conducted a 3-year reevaluation, as required by special education law. To assess his current behavioral and emotional functioning, the MDT obtained the CBCL from Mrs. Conner, TRFs from several of his ninth-grade teachers and his special education case manager, and the YSR from Kyle. The evaluation also included cognitive and achievement testing and interviews with Mrs. Conner, Kyle, and his teachers.

Figure 6.1 shows Kyle's scores on the CBCL problem scales at age 15 (solid line) and age 12 (broken line), based on Mrs. Conner's ratings. At age 15, Kyle's scores on the CBCL Withdrawn, Anxious/Depressed, Social Problems, Thought Problems, and Attention Problems scales were all considerably lower than at age 12. Normal range scores on six of the eight CBCL scales indicated substantial improvement in Kyle's function-

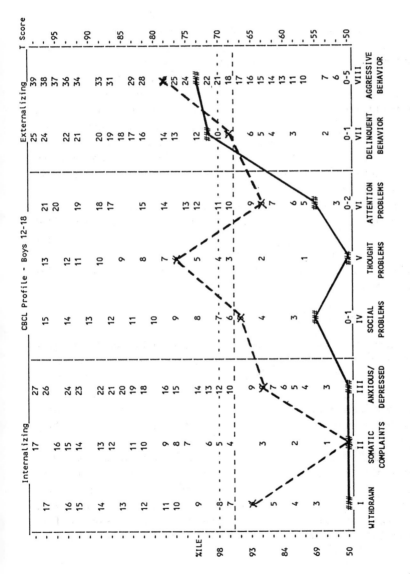

Figure 6.1. CBCL problem profiles for Kyle at age 15 (solid line) and age 12 (broken line).

151

ing in several areas, as did the 10-point drop in his Internalizing raw score from the clinical to the normal range. However, Kyle's scores on the Delinquent Behavior and Aggressive Behavior scales continued to indicate severe externalizing behaviors at age 15.

The TRF obtained from Kyle's special education case manager produced borderline clinical scores on all TRF syndromes except Thought Problems and Attention Problems. A TRF from Kyle's ninth-grade math teacher also produced borderline to clinical range scores on the Withdrawn, Social Problems, and Aggressive Behavior scales, whereas a TRF from his vocational education teacher produced normal range scores on all scales except Social Problems.

Figure 6.2 shows Kyle's scores on the YSR problem scales from his self-ratings at age 15 (solid line) and age 12 (broken line). At age 15, Kyle reported fewer problems on the YSR Withdrawn scale, suggesting that he viewed his social involvements more positively than at age 12. However, he reported more problems at age 15 on the YSR Thought Problems, Delinquent Behavior, and Aggressive Behavior scales. On the Thought Problems scale, Kyle reported that he couldn't get his mind off certain thoughts (living on his own outside the family), storing up things he doesn't need, and strange ideas (people are always against him), reflecting problems similar to those revealed by the SCICA at age 12. On the YSR Delinquent Behavior and Aggressive Behavior scales, Kyle's borderline scores suggested a greater willingness to acknowledge externalizing behavior at age 15 than at age 12.

Case Formulation for Kyle at Age 15

Kyle's case illustrates a complex pattern of internalizing and externalizing problems in an adolescent boy who had experienced many changes in his life circumstances. Ratings on the CBCL and TRF continued to produce high scores on the Delinquent Behavior and Aggressive Behavior scales at age 15, similar to those found at age 12, although there was a drop in his TRF Aggressive Behavior score. Coupled with his mother's reports of aggressive behavior as early as age 6, these findings documented the persistence of aggressive behavior from early childhood to adolescence. Kyle's long-term pattern was consistent with the stability of Aggressive Behavior syndrome scores found in longitudinal research reviewed in Chapter 3. At age 12, evidence from the multiaxial assessment of Kyle supported a *DSM-IV* diagnosis of CD, Childhood-Onset type, which continued to be appropriate at age 15. Although the empirically

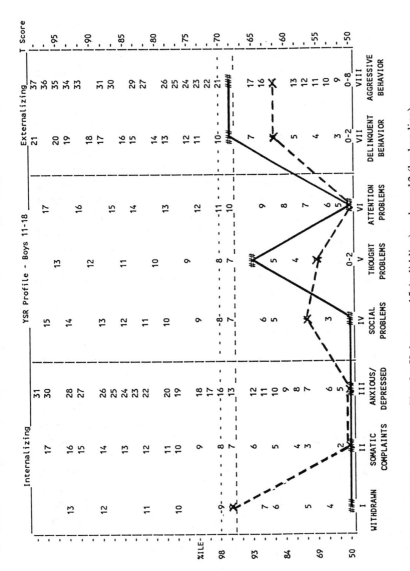

Figure 6.2. YSR problem profiles for Kyle at age 15 (solid line) and age 12 (broken line).

153

based measures were not designed specifically to make *DSM* diagnoses, item and scale scores on the Delinquent Behavior and Aggressive Behavior syndromes were consistent with CD behaviors reported during interviews with Kyle and his mother. In addition to externalizing problems, the age 15 TRF from the special education case manager produced borderline clinical scores on the Anxious/Depressed, Withdrawn, Somatic Complaints, and Social Problems scales. A TRF from Kyle's ninth-grade math teacher showed similar problems, but a TRF from his vocational education teacher showed a much more positive picture, with only the Social Problems scale reaching the borderline clinical range. At age 15, Kyle's CBCL also produced normal range scores on six scales, indicating an improvement in Kyle's functioning in several areas compared to his CBCL at age 12.

On the YSR, Kyle reported more problems on the Thought Problems, Delinquent Behavior, and Aggressive Behavior scales than he did at age 12, producing scores in the borderline clinical range on the latter two scales. His high scores on the two Externalizing scales were consistent with his age 15 CBCL and TRF. At age 12, Kyle's YSR scores had been markedly lower than his CBCL and TRF scores on all scales except Withdrawn, because he denied many problems reported by parents and teachers.

Despite the persistence of Kyle's externalizing behavior, the CBCL and YSR at age 15 suggested some improvement in his internalizing problems. In contrast, high scores for the Internalizing and Externalizing syndromes on two age 15 TRFs suggested that Kyle's school-based behavioral/emotional problems continued unabated. This justified behavioral interventions like those provided in his age 12 IEP, but adapted for older adolescents. Kyle's higher scores on the YSR at age 15 than at age 12 also indicated that he was now more willing to acknowledge thought problems, as well as aggressive and delinquent behavior, which might facilitate cognitive behavioral interventions involving his cooperation. Relatively low problem scores on the TRF completed by his vocational education teacher also indicated that Kyle functioned much better in courses geared toward job training and community-based skills. This was important to consider in designing an educational program that meshed with Kyle's strong work ethic and desire to become independent from his family.

Kyle's case illustrated persistent aggressive behavior with co-occurring emotional problems in an adolescent boy. We now turn to the case of Julie to illustrate the developmental course of emotional and conduct problems that do not include severe aggressive behavior.

CASE 4. JULIE:
AN ADOLESCENT ARRESTED FOR
DELINQUENT BEHAVIOR

After 14-year-old Julie Meyer was arrested for shoplifting, the juvenile court referred her to the local community mental health center (CMHC) for evaluation as part of their court diversion program for first offenders. Julie was an only child living with her adoptive parents, Susan and Richard Meyer, who had served as foster parents prior to adopting her. For her evaluation, the CMHC clinician interviewed Julie and Mrs. Meyer, obtained the CBCL from Mrs. Meyer, the YSR from Julie, and TRFs from two of Julie's eighth-grade teachers. Four years earlier, the state social service agency had also obtained a CBCL from Mrs. Meyer and a TRF from Julie's fourth-grade teacher to evaluate her functioning 6 months after she was placed with the Meyers as a foster child. To illustrate the developmental pattern of Julie's problems, we first summarize her history up to age 14 and then compare findings on the age 10 and age 14 CBCLs, TRFs, and YSR.

Julie's History to Age 14

Julie was the only child of Louise and Steven Boyd. The Boyds had a stormy and sometimes violent marriage that ended in divorce when Julie was 5 years old. After the divorce, Julie lived with her mother and visited her father on weekends. Both Mr. and Mrs. Boyd had histories of alcohol and drug abuse. Mrs. Boyd also suffered from bipolar disorder. Following their divorce, Mr. and Mrs. Boyd each had a series of unstable relationships, resulting in numerous changes in Julie's home environments. Julie was often left unsupervised while her mother was out with friends at night. When Julie was 10 years old, she was taken into state custody due to neglect by her mother and physical abuse by her father and her mother's boyfriend. She was then placed with Mr. and Mrs. Meyer as foster parents. During the first year of her foster placement, Julie continued to have supervised visits with her mother and father on alternating weekends. However, parental rights were eventually terminated, thereby opening the way for the Meyers to adopt Julie at age 12.

Mrs. Meyer reported that Julie had long been a moody and troubled child. When she was first placed in their foster home, she was sad, sullen, and irritable much of the time. She often retreated into herself when Mrs. Meyer tried to discuss her feelings. She also had few friends and seemed to prefer younger children. As she approached adolescence, Julie's mood swings decreased and she seemed more happier and more outgoing. Over the past year, however, Julie began associating with other kids whom Mrs. Meyer considered to be bad influences. Her new friends were often unsupervised at night and were known as troublemakers in the community. Mrs. Meyer became more concerned when Julie started staying out beyond her curfew and failed to report home on her whereabouts. Mrs. Meyer was also worried that Julie was becoming sexually active. When confronted about these issues, Julie often lied about her activities or refused to talk. One month prior to her referral to the CMHC, Julie was arrested for stealing a sweater from a local clothing store.

Parent Reports for Julie at Age 14 Versus Age 10

To provide a visual comparison of Julie's pattern of problems at two assessment points, Figure 6.3 shows her scores from the CBCL profiles obtained when she was referred to the CMHC at age 14 (solid line) and at age 10 (broken line), 6 months after her foster placement with Mr. and Mrs. Meyer. By plotting Julie's scores on the hand-scored version of the CBCL profile, we are able to display scores compared to the normative samples for ages 4 to 11 and ages 12 to 18 on the same profile. The item scores are omitted from Figure 6.3.

At age 14, Julie's CBCL profile showed a marked peak on the Delinquent Behavior scale, with a T score of 76. On this scale, Mrs. Meyer scored as *very true or often true* the items, *Doesn't seem to feel guilty after misbehaving, Lying or cheating, Prefers playing with older children,* and *Thinks about sex too much.* She scored as *somewhat or sometimes true* the items, *Hangs around with children who get in trouble, Steals at home,* and *Steals outside the home.* In contrast, Julie's score on the Aggressive Behavior scale was well within the normal range. Her scores on the remaining scales were also in the normal range, except for a borderline score for Withdrawn. On this scale, Mrs. Meyer endorsed six of the nine items, including, *Likes to be alone; Refuses to talk; Secretive, keeps things to herself; Sulks a lot; Underactive, slow moving, or lacks energy;* and *Withdrawn, doesn't get involved with others.*

In contrast to her age 14 score, Julie's age 10 score for Delinquent Behavior was much lower and well within the normal range for girls age 4 to 11. Mrs. Meyer reported only lacking guilt after misbehaving as *somewhat or sometimes true* at age 10. However, she endorsed many more items on the Withdrawn, Social Problems, and Attention Problems scales, producing scores in the borderline to clinical range. Julie's score on the

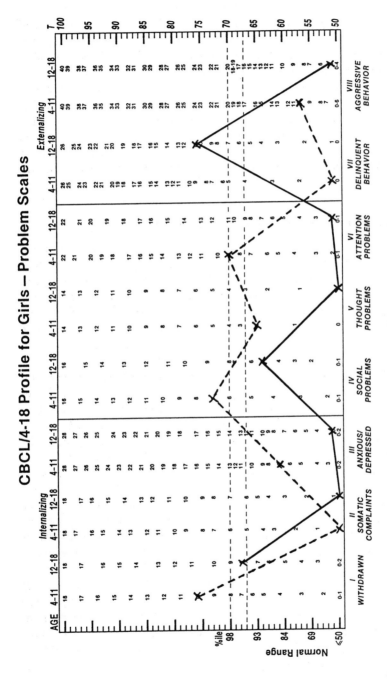

Figure 6.3. Hand-scored CBCL problem profiles for Julie at age 14 (solid line) and age 10 (broken line).

157

Withdrawn scale was similar to her age 14 score, whereas her scores on the Anxious/Depressed, Social Problems, Thought Problems, and Attention Problems scales were all higher at age 10 than at age 14. At age 10, Julie's CBCL Internalizing score was in the clinical range, but her Externalizing score was in the normal range. At age 14, this pattern was reversed, with her Externalizing score in the clinical range and her Internalizing score in the normal range. However, Julie's scores for Aggressive Behavior remained low at both ages.

Teacher Reports for Julie at Age 14 Versus Age 10

Figure 6.4 shows Julie's scores on the TRF profiles obtained from her eighth-grade English teacher at age 14 (solid line) and from her fourth-grade teacher at age 10 (broken line). At age 14, Julie's scores on all TRF scales fell in the normal range, with a pattern that was remarkably similar to her TRF profile pattern at age 10. Her moderately high scores on the Social Problems and Aggressive Behavior scales reflected poor peer relations, arguing, mood changes, stubbornness, and demands for attention, but very little physical aggression. Julie's teachers also reported several problems on the Anxious/Depressed scale, including occasional sadness, feeling unloved and worthless, and feeling that others were out to get her. Julie's scores on the Delinquent Behavior scale, however, were well within the normal range on both the age 10 and age 14 TRFs. At age 10, Julie's teacher reported that she sometimes lacked guilt after misbehaving, whereas at age 14, her teacher reported she was sometimes tardy, but both teachers scored all other items on the Delinquent Behavior scale as *not true*. At age 14, an additional TRF obtained from Julie's math teacher (not displayed in Figure 6.4) produced scores well within the normal range on all scales.

Direct Assessment of Julie at Age 14

Prior to her interview with the CMHC clinician, Julie completed the YSR. On the competence portion, Julie reported participating in field hockey and band at school, but otherwise had few hobbies or activities and no chores at home. As a result, her YSR Activities and total competence scores fell in the borderline range for girls age 11 to 18. Her score on the YSR Social scale was in the normal range, reflecting positive self-ratings of relationships with friends and family members, although she participated in no organized social groups or clubs.

Figure 6.5 (pp. 160-162) shows the computer-scored version of Julie's YSR problem profile, which had borderline to clinical range peaks on the

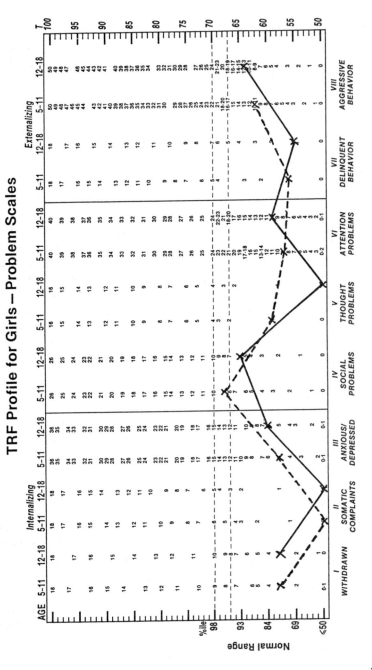

Figure 6.4. Hand-scored TRF problem profiles for Julie at age 14 (solid line) and age 10 (broken line).

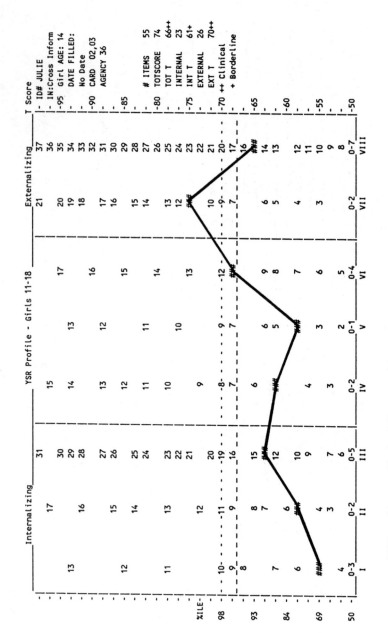

Figure 6.5. YSR problem profile for Julie at age 14.

160

WITHDRAWN	SOMATIC COMPLAINTS	ANXIOUS/ DEPRESSED	SOCIAL PROBLEMS	THOUGHT PROBLEMS	ATTENTION PROBLEMS	DELINQUENT BEHAVIOR	AGGRESSIVE BEHAVIOR	OTHER PROBS
1 42.Rather BeAlone	0 51. Dizzy	2 12.Lonely	2 1. Acts Young	2 9. Mind Off	1 1. Acts Young	2 26.NoGuilt	1 3. Argues	0 5. ActOppSex
2 54. Tired	2 54. Tired	1 14.Cries	0 11.Clings	0 40.Hears Things	1 8. Concen- trate	2 39.BadCompan	1 7. Brags	1 22.Disobey
1 56a.Aches	1 56a.Aches	1 18.HarmSelf*	1 25.NotGet Along	2 66.Repeats Acts	0 10.Sit Still	2 43.LieCheat	1 16.Mean	1 24.NotEat
0 65.Won't Talk	1 56b.Head- aches	0 31.FearDoBad	0 38.Teased	0 70.Sees Things	0 13.Con- fused	2 63.PrefOlder	0 19.DemAttn	2 29.Fears
1 69.Secret- ive	0 56c.Nausea	2 32.Perfect	1 48.Not Liked	1 83.Store Up*	2 17.Day- dream	0 67.RunAway	0 20.DestOwn	0 30.FearSchool
0 75.Shy	0 56d.Eye	0 33.Unloved	1 62.Clumsy	1 84.Strange Behav	2 41.Impul- sive	0 72.SetFires	0 21.DestOthr	0 36.GetHurt
1 102.Under- active	0 56e.Skin	1 34.OutToGet	0 64.Prefers Young	0 85.Strange Ideas	1 45.Nervous	0 81.StealHome	0 23.DisobSchl	0 44.BiteNail
1 103.Sad	1 56f.Stomach	0 35.Worthless	0 111.With- drawn*	4 TOTAL	0 61.Poor School	2 82.StealOut	0 27.Jealous	0 46.Twitch
1 111.With- drawn	0 56g.Vomit	1 45.Nervous	5 TOTAL	58 T SCORE	1 62.Clumsy	1 90.Swears	0 37.Fights	0 47.Nightmares
5 TOTAL	5 TOTAL	1 50.Fearful	61 T SCORE	49 CLIN T	10 TOTAL	1 101.Truant	0 57.Attacks	1 53.EatTooMuch
55 T SCORE	58 T SCORE	0 52.Guilty	52 CLIN T		67 T SCORE	0 105.AlcDrugs	1 68.Screams	1 55.OverWeight
45 CLIN T	49 CLIN T	2 71.SelfConsc			56 CLIN T	11 TOTAL	2 74.ShowOff	0 56h.OtherPhys
		0 89.Suspicious				75 T SCORE	2 86.Stubborn	0 58.PickSkin
		1 91.Think				65 CLIN T	2 87.MoodChnge	0 76.Sleepless
		Suicide*					2 93.TalkMuch	2 77.SleepMore
		1 103.Sad					1 94.Teases	0 79.SpeechProb
		1 112.Worries					1 95.Temper	2 96.ThinkSex
		14 TOTAL					0 97.Threaten	0 99.TooNeat
		64 T SCORE					1 104.Loud	0 100.SleepProb
		52 CLIN T					15 TOTAL	0 110.WishOpSex
							65 T SCORE	
							53 CLIN T	

*Items not on Cross-Informant Construct

Not in Total Problem Score
0 2.Allergy 0 4.Asthma

Profile Type:	WTHDR	SOMAT	SOCIAL	DEL-AGG	YSR Soc	Delinq
ICC:	-.633	-.491	-.266	.583**	-.287	.052

** Significant ICC with profile type

Figure 6.5. (Continued)

161

Attention Problems and Delinquent Behavior scales. On the Attention Problems scale, Julie reported many more problems than did her mother or teachers, including difficulty concentrating, daydreaming, restlessness, and impulsivity. On the Delinquent Behavior scale, Julie acknowledged many of the same problems reported by Mrs. Meyer, including stealing outside the home. In addition, she reported sometimes being truant, which was not reported by Mrs. Meyer or her teachers. She did not report using alcohol or drugs. Julie's scores on the remaining six YSR scales were all in the normal range, although her score for Aggressive Behavior exceeded the 93rd percentile. On the Aggressive Behavior scale, Julie reported problems such as arguing, screaming, stubbornness, and mood changes, but no physical aggression toward people or property. On the Thought Problems scale, Julie reported that she could not get her mind off certain thoughts (boys and friends), storing up things she doesn't need, and strange behavior. She also scored as *very true or often true* the item, *I think about sex too much,* and as *somewhat or sometimes true* the items, *I deliberately try to hurt or kill myself* and *I think about killing myself.*

During the SCICA, Julie openly discussed personal issues and problems. She reported that before seventh grade, she was shy, felt unaccepted, and was often teased by other kids in school. She kept mostly to herself and seldom invited kids to her house. When she entered seventh grade, she joined band and other school activities that expanded her social contacts. Later that year, she began hanging around with two girls who were disliked by her parents. These new friendships led to arguments with her parents, particularly when she stayed out late and failed to tell her parents where she was going. She reported that her friends sometimes dared her to take things from local stores (e.g., cigarettes, candy, or pens), and that she sometimes skipped school with them, but neither her teachers nor her parents knew about these incidents. Julie also began dating in seventh grade. By age 14, Julie had had several sexual experiences with three different boyfriends. She found some of these experiences disturbing because she did not know how to say no to boys. She said she often thought about sex and hoped someday to be happily married with children. She reported that when she was younger, an older stepbrother in her father's home had made sexual advances, but she denied having been sexually molested.

At age 14, Julie was still angry at her biological parents, who in her words, "abandoned her." She felt close to her adoptive parents but had trouble trusting them. When asked about her scores on the YSR items concerning suicide, Julie reported that she sometimes feels there is no point to living and had thought about taking overdoses of aspirin when she felt depressed. However, Julie denied having any intentions or specific plans for suicide.

When asked about her court charges, Julie reported that she and her girlfriend tried on sweaters in a clothing store and then walked out without paying for them. Julie was caught by police just outside the store, but her girlfriend escaped undetected. Julie was worried about what would happen to her now that she had been caught shoplifting. She described the court proceedings as frightening and felt guilty that she had disappointed her adoptive parents. She was eager to talk with a counselor about her problems and particularly wanted help in dealing with peer pressure in the future.

Cognitive and Physical Assessment

Julie's assessment at age 14 focused primarily on her behavioral and emotional functioning, particularly the delinquent behavior that led to the court diversion. However, the CMHC clinician administered the WISC-III to assess her cognitive strengths and weaknesses. Julie obtained a verbal IQ of 96, a performance IQ of 111, and a full scale IQ of 102, placing her in the average range. Her scores were average to above average on all WISC-III subtests, with the exception of a below average score for short-term auditory attention. Her eighth-grade teachers also reported average academic performance, although Julie sometimes failed to complete assignments on time. Julie's teachers reported that she demonstrated good math skills when she applied herself and was talented in band and field hockey. They described her as a pleasant and cooperative student but noted that she sometimes showed unexplained mood swings and seemed unsure of herself in social groups.

A recent exam by Julie's pediatrician indicated normal physical health and normal pubertal development with menses beginning at age 13. The pediatrician noted, however, that Julie was self-conscious about being examined by a male physician and refused to discuss her sexual development. At Mrs. Meyer's request, the pediatrician referred Julie to a female gynecologist for a follow-up visit and subsequent discussion of safe-sex practices.

Case Formulation for Julie at Age 14

Like Kyle in the preceding case illustration, Julie had problems at age 14 that were consistent with a *DSM-IV* diagnosis of CD. The CBCL and

YSR, plus interviews with Julie and her adoptive mother, provided evidence for behaviors required for a diagnosis of CD, including having stolen items of nontrivial value, often lying, and often staying out late at night despite parental prohibition. Julie also reported occasionally being truant from school, but for CD, *DSM-IV* requires onset of truancy before age 13 and a greater frequency than reported by Julie. Her sexual activity was also of great concern to Julie's mother, but promiscuity is not among the criteria for CD. Julie's clinical range scores on the Delinquent Behavior scales of the CBCL and YSR supported the CD diagnosis. In contrast to Kyle, however, Julie did not show significant conduct problems at earlier ages, as gleaned from accounts of her history from Mrs. Meyer and normal range scores on the CBCL and TRF Externalizing scales at age 10. Lacking CD behaviors prior to age 10, Julie qualified for a *DSM-IV* diagnosis of CD, Adolescent-Onset type.

The contrast between Julie and Kyle is also remarkable for the differences in their aggressive behavior. Although, at age 14, Julie and one teacher reported arguing, stubbornness, showing off, and mood changes, her CBCL, TRF, and YSR Aggressive Behavior scores were all in the normal range. Julie's age 10 CBCL and TRF also produced normal range scores for Aggressive Behavior. Julie's conduct problems thus consisted mainly of nonaggressive delinquent behavior, whereas Kyle's problems included both aggressive and delinquent behaviors. As indicated in Chapter 3, the *DSM-IV* diagnosis of CD lacks the distinction between aggressive versus nonaggressive CD that was made by *DSM-III*. Yet in Julie's case, as in Kyle's, such a distinction was important to consider in planning appropriate interventions.

Cross-informant comparisons of the CBCL, two TRFs, and YSR obtained for Julie at age 14 showed average agreement between Julie and her mother, as indicated by the Q correlations between their scores. Julie and Mrs. Meyer agreed in their ratings of similar items on the Delinquent Behavior syndrome, as well as several items on the Social Problem syndrome. In addition, Mrs. Meyer reported problems on the Withdrawn syndrome, consistent with her earlier ratings of Julie at age 10. Julie's continuing problems in peer relations contributed to her self-acknowledged attempts to win friends via delinquent behavior. During the clinical interview, Julie described incidents of shoplifting, skipping school, and violating her curfew at the behest of friends. She also reported sexual activities motivated by desire for acceptance, even though she was troubled and frightened by the sexual advances of her boyfriends. Julie's case thus illustrates the strong influence of socially deviant peers on adolescent onset delinquency, as described by Moffitt (1993).

In addition to delinquent behavior, Julie reported many problems on the YSR Attention Problems syndrome, including difficulty concentrating, daydreaming, restlessness, and impulsive behavior. Her mother also reported attention problems on the CBCL at age 10, but not at age 14, whereas teachers reported minimal attention problems on the TRF at both ages. These cross-informant variations suggested that Julie's self-reported attention problems were associated more with fluctuations in her emotional states than with ADHD. Julie's score on the YSR Anxious/Depressed scale was also notable, even though it did not reach the clinical range. On this scale, Julie endorsed 11 of the 16 items, including feeling lonely and sad, attempting to harm herself, and thinking about suicide. The clinical interview further revealed unresolved feelings of anger and sadness about her past history and her struggles for acceptance by peers. Although Julie appeared to be in no immediate danger of harming herself, her vulnerability to mood changes and feelings of hopelessness warranted careful monitoring.

Despite her emotional problems and delinquent behavior, Julie manifested several strengths. Her foster placement and subsequent adoption by Mr. and Mrs. Meyer gave her a supportive, stable home environment. The adolescent onset of Julie's delinquent behavior reflected peer influences that were amenable to change, rather than a persistent pattern of antisocial behavior. Interventions to change Julie's peer group and to improve her social coping skills had good prospects for success. Julie's frightened and remorseful reaction to being arrested for shoplifting, coupled with her desire for counseling, were also positive signs of her desire to change. In addition, Julie's teachers reported good academic progress and growing participation in school activities, while cognitive testing demonstrated average to above-average ability. Julie thus presented many personal, cognitive, and academic strengths on which to capitalize in designing interventions.

Interventions and Outcomes for Julie

Because her arrest for shoplifting was a first offense, Julie was eligible for a court diversion program that required counseling plus 40 hours of community service. She began weekly individual therapy with the CMHC counselor. Therapy sessions focused on (a) improving self-esteem, (b) developing social coping strategies and assertiveness, (c) understanding sexuality and safe-sex practices, and (d) coping with feelings of anger and sadness. The counselor also met with Julie and her parents to develop a behavioral contract regarding household rules, curfews, and activities with friends. Mr. and Mrs. Meyer, in collaboration with school staff, increased their efforts to involve Julie in organized social activities. She continued to participate in band and team sports at school and joined an after-school club. The school staff also encouraged Julie to join the stage crew for the eighth-grade school play. These activities introduced Julie to several new friends, who served as better role models than her former friends. To meet her community service obligation, Julie worked after school hours twice a week in a local hospital.

To evaluate Julie's progress at age 15, the juvenile court diversion program obtained the CBCL from Mrs. Meyer, the YSR from Julie, and a TRF from the high school teacher who knew her best. The results were shared with the CMHC clinician, who continued to work with Julie and her parents. The CBCL and YSR profiles both showed marked improvements on the Delinquent Behavior and Externalizing scales, where Julie's scores dropped into the normal range. Her scores on the TRF scales also remained in the normal range. Thus, a year after Julie's arrest at age 14, the empirically based measures at age 15 documented significant reductions in her delinquent behavior. On the YSR, however, she continued to report anxiety, depression, and somatic complaints, resulting in a borderline clinical score for Internalizing. Because of these persistent emotional problems, the CMHC continued to provide counseling services to Julie and her family as needed.

SUMMARY

This chapter illustrated multiaxial empirically based assessment of adolescents. Like many adolescents, both Kyle and Julie manifested conduct problems that qualified for a *DSM-IV* diagnosis of CD. However, the kinds of conduct problems that they manifested, their developmental course, and their likely prognosis were quite different.

As documented by empirically based assessment at several ages, Kyle manifested a persistent pattern of aggressive behavior in multiple contexts. He occasionally engaged in more covert delinquent behavior as well. Kyle's strengths included skills in sports, a strong work ethic, a growing willingness to acknowledge his problems, and motivation to become independent from his family. He was also responsive to some of the interventions that were designed to improve his behavior. However, his recurrent aggressive behavior despite various environmental changes was consistent with longitudinal evidence that high scores on the Aggressive Behavior syndrome tend to be quite stable over the course of development. On the other hand, longitudinal research also shows that, for some youths, high scores on the Aggressive Behavior syndrome are succeeded in young adulthood by high scores on a syndrome designated as Shows Off (Achenbach et al., 1995c). The Shows Off syndrome includes the socially intrusive behaviors of the pre-adult Aggressive Behavior syndrome, but not its overtly aggressive behaviors. Although Kyle's long-term prognosis is not favorable, it is possible that his most destructive aggressive behaviors will subside while his socially intrusive behaviors persist. In any event, continuing interventions are apt to be needed throughout adolescence to maximize control over Kyle's aggressive behavior while helping him develop vocational and academic skills necessary for adult adaptation.

Like Kyle, Julie qualified for a diagnosis of CD. This is not surprising in view of the deviant behavior of Julie's biological parents and her stressful childhood. However, Julie's conduct problems were primarily the nonaggressive behaviors of the Delinquent Behavior syndrome, and they began in adolescence, primarily as efforts to gain acceptance from peers. The love and support provided by Julie's adoptive parents, her lack of overtly aggressive behavior, her remorse for her delinquent behavior, and the decline in this behavior by age 15 all boded well for her future development.

Although both adolescents qualified for CD diagnoses, Julie's empirically based profiles revealed patterns that were quite different from Kyle's. Based both on longitudinal research reviewed in Chapter 3 and on the specifics of each case, Julie's conduct problems appeared to reflect more transient developmental issues and to be more susceptible to environmental influences than Kyle's.

7

ILLUSTRATIONS OF SPECIAL ASSESSMENT NEEDS

In previous chapters, we illustrated empirically based assessment of children and adolescents with a variety of problems, including attention deficits, conduct disorders, and affective disorders. This chapter presents applications of empirically based assessment to a mentally retarded boy with disturbed thinking and behavior problems that led to placement in a residential treatment center. We then turn to the cases of three boys whose learning and behavioral problems at age 6 led to an intervention for their entire first-grade class. These three boys were introduced in the first edition of this book. By returning to their cases, we demonstrate how data from the pre-1991 editions of the CBCL and TRF profiles can be rescored on the 1991 profiles. Once pre-1991 data have been entered into computer files, they can be scored again using the 1991 CBCL and TRF computer programs or the cross-informant program.

CASE 5. MICHAEL:
A BOY IN A RESIDENTIAL
TREATMENT CENTER

Michael Granger was the youngest of six children in a low-income family. His parents divorced when he was 2 years old, leaving his mother with sole responsibility for the children. As Michael grew older, Mrs. Granger experienced increasing difficulty dealing with his oppositional and aggressive behavior. She also worried about Michael's growing preoccupation with war and violence. Despite his mother's admonitions, Michael insisted on watching violent TV shows and was fascinated with guns, knives, and military weapons. Michael's pretend play was violent as well. Sometimes Mrs. Granger wondered whether Michael could distinguish fantasy from reality, especially when he dressed as a Japanese ninja warrior and demanded that family members bow to him and feign fear when he attacked them. Despite being Caucasian, Michael was convinced that his father and grandfather had been ninjas.

When Michael became angry at his mother or siblings, he often threatened them with toy guns or toy knives. At least once a week, he threw temper tantrums and destroyed objects and furniture in the home. These incidents provoked severe physical punishments from Mrs. Granger, but punishment had little effect on Michael's behavior. Even with home-based services from a state agency, Mrs. Granger was often unable to control Michael's behavior.

At age 9, Michael assaulted his mother with a kitchen knife. After a frantic phone call from Mrs. Granger, the police and a social worker removed Michael from the home. He was placed in a residential treatment center for observation and evaluation. The evaluation indicated mild to moderate mental retardation and intermittent psychotic thought processes. On the recommendation of the assessment team, Michael was admitted to the center's residential program, where he was housed in a group home with five other children and two full-time child care workers. A social worker supervised visits by Michael to his family on weekends. Michael's treatment program included a structured behavior management program in the group home, weekly individual therapy, and medication with haloperidol (Haldol) to reduce aggressiveness and psychotic thought processes. Michael also attended the treatment center's school, where he received special education, speech and language services, and social skills training. The school used a behavior modification program that was coordinated with the group home program.

At age 11, Michael moved from the group home to a therapeutic foster home operated by the treatment center. He continued to visit his biological family at least once a month, although his mother was still unable to manage his behavior without help. From age 9 to 12, Michael advanced from fourth to sixth grade in the center's school. At age 12, Michael was reassessed to evaluate his progress and to plan future treatment. His treatment team needed to decide whether to move Michael from the foster home to his mother's home and from the center's school to a public school, because he was approaching the center's age limit and his state was committed to mainstreaming.

The multiaxial assessment at age 9 had included the CBCL from Mrs. Granger when Michael was first placed in residential treatment, plus a

CBCL from the child care worker and a TRF from the center's teacher 2 months after his initial placement. The age 12 assessment included a CBCL from Michael's foster parent, TRFs from two sixth-grade teachers in the center's school, and a YSR from Michael, plus empirically based measures of social skills and adaptive behavior. At ages 9 and 12, the Woodcock Johnson Psychoeducational Battery-Revised (WJPB-R; Woodcock & Johnson, 1989) was used to evaluate Michael's cognitive ability and academic achievement. To illustrate Michael's functioning over the course of his treatment, we will compare findings from his age 9 and age 12 CBCLs, TRFs, and WJPB-R. We will also summarize his age 12 scores on the YSR and social skills and adaptive measures.

Parent Reports at Ages 9 and 12

Figure 7.1 shows Michael's CBCL profiles from ratings by three parent figures: his mother at age 9, at the beginning of his placement in the treatment center (solid line); a child care worker at age 9, 2 months after his placement (dotted line); and his foster parent at age 12 (broken line). All three CBCLs yielded clinical range scores on the Social Problems scale, reflecting immature behavior and difficulty relating to peers, and on the Thought Problems scale, reflecting disturbed thinking. Mrs. Granger and the child care worker both endorsed obsessions, strange ideas, and strange behavior, whereas the child care worker also endorsed repetitive acts. Like Mrs. Granger, the child care worker noted that Michael could not get his mind off being a ninja warrior, often pretended to be a ninja, and fabricated stories about ninja escapades with his father and grandfather. The child care worker also reported that Michael seldom made eye contact, frequently wet the bed, and sometimes masturbated in public.

Michael's age 9 CBCL from his mother had additional clinical range peaks on the Withdrawn, Anxious/Depressed, Attention Problems, Delinquent Behavior, and Aggressive Behavior scales. The CBCL from the child care worker also yielded borderline to clinical range scores on the Withdrawn, Attention Problems, and Delinquent Behavior scales. However, Michael's score on the Aggressive Behavior scale was much lower than on his mother's CBCL, indicating that his aggressive behavior was better controlled in the residential center than it had been at home.

At age 12, the CBCL from Michael's foster parent indicated substantial improvements in several areas, with normal range scores on the With-

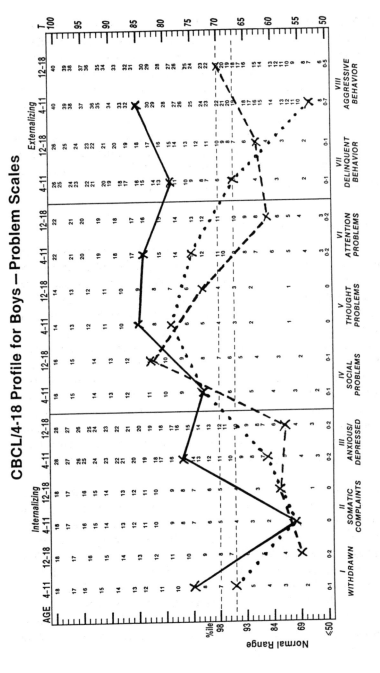

Figure 7.1. CBCL problem profiles for Michael scored at age 9 by his mother (solid line) and child care worker (dotted line) and at age 12 by his foster parent (broken line).

drawn, Anxious/Depressed, Attention Problems, and Delinquent Behavior scales. However, Michael's score on the Aggressive Behavior scale was in the borderline range, indicating more aggressive behavior in the foster home at age 12 than in the group home at age 9. Michael's foster parent endorsed as *very true or often true* arguing, bragging, showing off, and talking too much, and as *somewhat or sometimes true,* problems such as destroying other people's things, disobeying at home and school, physically attacking people, and temper tantrums. On the Thought Problems scale, the foster parent reported obsessions with weapons and the military, repetitive actions, and strange ideas that suggested poor reality testing.

On the CBCL competence scales at age 12, Michael scored well within the normal range on the Activities scale, but in the clinical range on the Social scale. His score on the Activities scale was much higher at age 12 than it had been at age 9 on his mother's CBCL. Michael's foster parent reported that he played on a basketball team at the treatment center in addition to enjoying bike riding and fishing. He also performed his assigned chores in the foster home at an average level. However, Michael was not involved in any organized social groups and continued to have problems getting along with his foster parent and biological family.

To provide an assessment of Michael's social skills and adaptive behavior, his foster parent completed the Social Skills Rating System (SSRS; Gresham & Elliott, 1990) and the Comprehensive Test of Adaptive Behavior (CTAB; Adams, 1984). The SSRS indicated average social skills compared to norms for boys in Grades 7 to 12. On the SSRS subscales, Michael scored in the average range for cooperation and responsibility, but below average for assertion and self-control. On the CTAB, the foster parent rated Michael's self-help skills related to toileting, grooming, dressing, and eating and his home-living skills related to activities and chores in various areas of the household and yard. Compared to the CTAB normative sample of 12-year-old boys, Michael scored below average for both self-help and home-living skills, with scores falling below the 5th percentile. However, compared to mentally retarded boys in nonschool settings, Michael scored above average, with scores at the 85th percentile for self-help and the 80th percentile for home living. He also scored in the average range for mentally retarded boys in less restrictive school settings, with scores at the 45th percentile for self-help and 30th percentile for home living. The results on the CTAB thus indicated that Michael's adaptive behavior was below average for boys with normal cognitive ability, but average to above average for mentally retarded boys.

Teacher Reports at Ages 9 and 12

Figure 7.2 shows Michael's scores on TRFs obtained at age 9 from his fourth-grade teacher (solid line) and at age 12 from two sixth-grade teachers (broken and dotted lines). All three TRFs yielded borderline to clinical range scores on the Withdrawn, Anxious/Depressed, Social Problems, and Attention Problems scales. At age 9, the TRF yielded normal range scores on the Delinquent Behavior and Aggressive Behavior scales, in contrast to borderline to clinical scores on these scales at age 12. Thus, even though he remained in the treatment center's school, Michael's classroom externalizing behavior increased substantially from age 9 to age 12. Michael also showed more attention problems and more thought problems in school at age 12 than he did at age 9. Both sixth-grade teachers reported obsessions, fears, repetitive acts, strange behavior, and strange ideas. They agreed with the foster parent that Michael continued to have trouble distinguishing between fantasy and reality and that he retreated into fantasy when he was upset. They also reported that he sometimes wore military costumes to school and used military gestures (e.g., saluting), sucked his thumb in class, and voiced fears about people being out to get him.

The SSRS completed by Michael's sixth-grade teachers yielded average scores for total social skills, assertion, and self-control, but a below average score for cooperation. Despite these positive scores, Michael's teachers reported that he continued to have difficulty in reasoning about social problems and in controlling his temper outbursts, which often led to removal from the classroom. Nevertheless, the teachers felt that Michael responded very well to the behavior management program in the classroom, often earning up to 80% of the possible points for special privileges and other reinforcers.

Cognitive Assessment at Ages 9 and 12

The WJPB-R was administered at ages 9 and 12 to assess Michael's cognitive ability and academic achievement. At age 9, Michael's standard score of 58 indicated below-average cognitive ability. Michael also scored below-average on all the WJPB-R achievement tests, with standard scores from 40 to 67. The results indicated mild to moderate retardation, with cognitive ability and academic achievement 2 to 3 years below his chronological age and grade placement.

At age 12, the WJPB-R showed some improvement in Michael's cognitive and academic functioning, with a cognitive ability score of 68 and

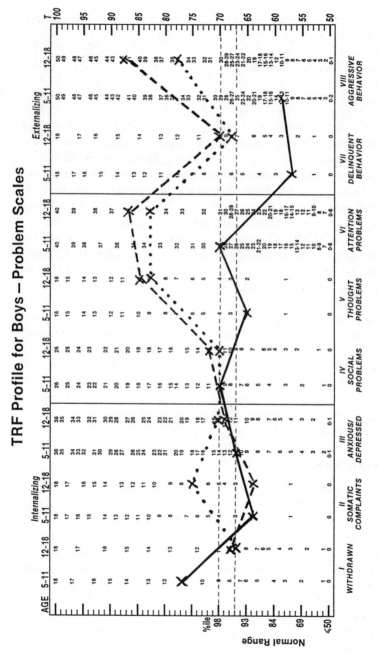

Figure 7.2. TRF problem profiles for Michael scored at age 9 by his fourth-grade teacher (solid line) and at age 12 by two sixth-grade teachers (dotted and broken lines).

achievement test scores from 50 to 70. The WJPB-R subtest scores indicated improvement in visual processing and reading compared to scores at age 9. However, Michael's ability and achievement performance remained 2 to 4 years below his chronological age and grade placement.

Michael's Self-Reports at Age 12

Because of Michael's poor reading skills, a teacher assisted him in completing the YSR. The teacher explained the YSR and read each item aloud to Michael. Michael then marked the appropriate response for each competence and problem item and wrote in his answers for open-ended items. The teacher reported that Michael appeared to understand the YSR questions and to give honest answers. The YSR profile yielded normal range scores on the Activities and Social scales. Michael reported interests in football, basketball, roller blading, and several other activities, and he listed the same household chores reported by his foster parent. He reported belonging to no social organizations but said he had four or more friends whom he saw regularly after school hours. All Michael's friends attended the treatment center school.

Michael also obtained normal range scores on all the YSR problem scales. However, he did report many problems on the Somatic Complaints scale, including dizziness, feeling tired, headaches, skin problems, stomachaches, and vomiting, yielding a score above the 90th percentile. On the Social Problems scale, Michael reported being too dependent on adults, getting teased, and not being liked. On the Aggressive Behavior scale, he reported arguing, physically attacking people, temper tantrums, talking too much, and being loud.

Summary of Michael

Michael illustrates empirically based assessment of a boy with mild to moderate mental retardation, disordered thought processes, and a propensity toward violent behavior. He met *DSM-IV* diagnostic criteria for mental retardation and CD. At age 9, CBCLs completed by Michael's mother and a child care worker, plus a TRF from his fourth-grade teacher, all yielded borderline to clinical range scores on the Withdrawn, Social Problems, and Attention Problems scales. The CBCL from Michael's mother also yielded clinical range scores on the Aggressive Behavior and Delinquent Behavior scales. After his admission to the residential program, Michael's antisocial and aggressive behavior decreased substantially, as evidenced by normal range scores on the CBCL and TRF Delinquent Behavior and Aggressive Behavior scales. However, Michael continued to obtain high scores on the CBCL Thought Problems scale, as he did prior to residential placement.

After 2 years in the treatment center's group home, Michael was moved to a therapeutic foster home and continued attending the school at the center. When Michael was 12, his treatment team needed to decide whether to return him to his biological family and a public school. The CBCL completed by Michael's foster parent indicated improvement on the Anxious/Depressed, Attention Problems, and Delinquent Behavior scales. Although Michael's borderline score on the Aggressive Behavior scale was also lower than on his mother's CBCL at age 9, it was much higher than his score on the CBCL at age 9 after 2 months in the treatment center's group home. TRFs from Michael's sixth-grade teachers yielded even higher scores for Aggressive Behavior, indicating that Michael was again showing severe aggression in school.

At age 12, Michael also obtained borderline to clinical scores on the CBCL and TRF Social Problems and Thought Problems scales, suggesting an emerging schizotypical personality disorder and/or psychosis. Although Michael reported fewer problems on the YSR, he did endorse somatic complaints, social problems, thought problems, and some aggressive behavior, indicating awareness of some of the problems reported by other informants.

Cognitive and achievement testing yielded below average scores on most WJPB-R scales, indicating mild to moderate mental retardation, which further complicated Michael's case. A 10-point increase in the WJPB-R cognitive ability score from age 9 to 12 suggested cognitive gains, but Michael continued to score 2 to 4 years below his agemates. The age 12 TRFs also showed severe attention problems in school, probably reflecting Michael's cognitive limitations. The CBCL Activities scale and measures of adaptive behavior and social skills produced more positive pictures of Michael's functioning, especially compared to mentally retarded boys. The adaptive measures suggested that Michael had adequate self-help skills and could participate appropriately in recreational and household activities under supervision.

The comprehensive assessment of Michael at age 12 warranted a guarded prognosis for his future. His cognitive limitations and severe aggressive behavior, coupled with disturbed thinking, continued to justify structured programs for behavior management, as well as mental health and special education services. Although Michael's mother and siblings remained involved with him, they agreed with the treatment team that out-of-home placement and special education continued to be appropriate for him.

CASE 6. TYRONE, LANCE, AND GERALD: A CLASSROOM INTERVENTION FOR DISRUPTIVE BEHAVIOR

Tyrone, Lance, and Gerald illustrate how the empirically based measures can be used to assess problems amenable to group interventions and to evaluate the outcomes of such interventions. Each of the boys was referred to the school psychologist by his first-grade teacher because of disruptive behavior and learning problems. After 2 months in first grade, Lance's teacher became concerned about his difficulty with basic skills and his confusion in class. She reported that Lance had difficulty understanding directions and was easily frustrated by schoolwork. He often cried in class and sometimes ripped up his papers when he could not do them correctly. Lance had poor relations with peers, was clumsy, and acted young for his age. To address these problems, Lance's teacher asked the school psychologist to observe his classroom behavior and to consult on appropriate accommodations.

Within the same month, the teacher also requested consultation regarding Tyrone and Gerald, who were inattentive, disruptive, and more aggressive than Lance. Like Lance, both boys often talked out of turn, disturbed other children, and failed to complete their schoolwork. Although Tyrone seemed intellectually capable, he was easily frustrated by the tedious aspects of schoolwork, refused to do his assignments, and threw temper tantrums in class. Tyrone also fought with other children on the playground, resulting in frequent trips to the principal's office. Gerald seemed moody and uninterested in school and argued a lot with the teacher. All three boys demanded a lot of attention, which the teacher felt was unfair to other students in the class.

To obtain a standardized, comprehensive assessment of their school problems, the school psychologist asked the teacher to complete the TRF on each boy. She then contacted each boy's mother to explain the teacher's concerns and request the CBCL. By comparing their TRF and CBCL profiles, the school psychologist could judge whether each boy's problems were restricted to the school setting or were broader in scope. The empirically based measures, plus additional information from parent and teacher interviews and classroom observations, were used to design interventions.

Teacher Reports at Time 1

On the TRFs completed for their initial assessment (Time 1), all three boys obtained low ratings for academic performance and total adaptive functioning. Their total problem and Externalizing scores were in the borderline to clinical range, indicating severe problems compared to normative samples. Gerald also obtained a borderline clinical score for Internalizing, indicating emotional problems as well as externalizing problems. Figure 7.3 displays the boys' patterns of problems superimposed onto one computer-scored TRF profile. All three boys had peaks on the TRF Social Problems and Attention Problems scales, with scores ranging from the 90th to 98th percentile. Tyrone and Gerald also scored in the borderline to clinical range for Aggressive Behavior. Reports of strange ideas for Tyrone and obsessional thoughts for Lance yielded scores just below the borderline range on the Thought Problems scale.

Parent Reports at Time 1

As shown in Figure 7.4, the three boys obtained different patterns of problems on the CBCLs completed by their mothers. Each boy had relatively high peaks on Attention Problems, consistent with the teacher's ratings on the TRF. High scores on the Social Problems scale for Lance and Gerald and on the Aggressive Behavior scale for Tyrone were also consistent with the teacher's ratings. However, compared to the teacher, Tyrone's mother reported more problems on the Withdrawn scale, whereas Lance's mother reported more problems on the Withdrawn, Somatic Complaints, Delinquent Behavior, and Aggressive Behavior scales. Gerald's CBCL indicated the fewest problems, including a much lower score for Aggressive Behavior than on the TRF. Cross-informant correlations indicated average to above-average parent-teacher agreement for each boy.

Cognitive Assessment at Time 1

Because all the boys were experiencing learning problems, the school MDT obtained parental permission to assess their cognitive ability and achievement to determine whether they needed special education or

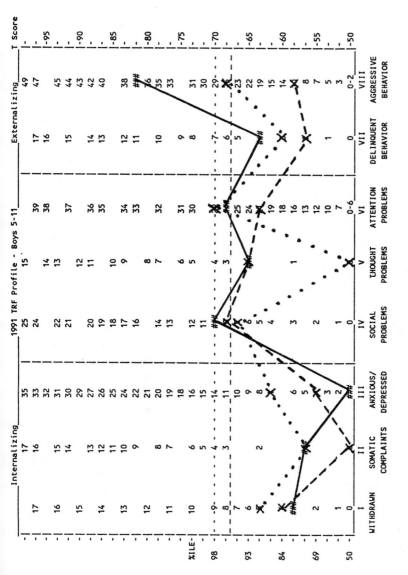

Figure 7.3. Time 1 TRF problem profiles for Tyrone (solid line), Lance (broken line), and Gerald (dotted line).

179

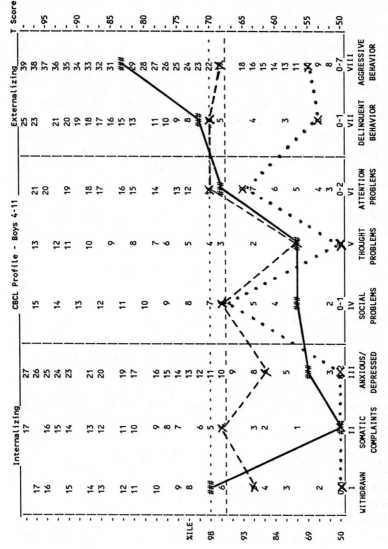

Figure 7.4. Time 1 CBCL problem profiles for Tyrone (solid line), Lance (broken line), and Gerald (dotted line).

remedial instruction. The McCarthy Scales of Children's Abilities (McCarthy, 1972) indicated average intelligence for all three boys. However, Lance scored below-average on tests of abstract verbal reasoning, auditory attention span, and fine and gross motor skills. Additional testing for Lance indicated below-average expressive language and reading achievement. Tyrone and Gerald both scored in the average range on achievement tests.

Direct Assessment at Time 1

To directly assess their school behavior, the school psychologist used the DOF to rate each boy's behavior on three occasions in the classroom. The DOF produced low on-task scores and high problem scores for all three boys, thus corroborating the teacher's reports on the TRF. The boys were on-task only 35% of the time, compared to 95% for two control boys in the same class. Tyrone, Lance, and Gerald all scored in the clinical range on the DOF Externalizing and Hyperactive scales. Tyrone also scored in the clinical range on the DOF Attention Demanding and Aggressive scales. The psychologist noted that all three boys were easily distracted, inattentive, and out of their seats much of the time. They also refused to cooperate in classroom routines and often argued with the teacher about the rules. The teacher had to repeat directions for each of them and remind them to get their pencils, crayons, papers, or books for the lesson.

Interventions for Tyrone, Lance, and Gerald

The TRF and DOF clearly indicated severe problems that warranted interventions in the school setting. However, the boys' mothers were concerned that the boys not be singled out from the rest of their first-grade class. The teacher and school psychologist agreed to try a token economy program for the entire class, because other children in the class were also inattentive and disruptive.

As a first step, the teacher and psychologist defined four target behaviors: getting ready for work on time; raising hand to talk; working quietly in seat; and finishing work on time. They then planned 5 days to initiate the program. On the first day, the teacher discussed the target behaviors with the class during circle time and demonstrated each behavior. To facilitate the discussion, the teacher created a laminated poster listing the four behaviors, which served as a daily reminder at the front of the classroom. The children all agreed that these behaviors were important parts of their "jobs" in school.

On the second day, the teacher explained how each student could earn one token for performing each of the target behaviors during three segments of the day: morning to recess; recess to lunch; and lunch to dismissal. This meant each child could earn up to 12 tokens per day. Paper pennies were provided as the tokens. As an art project, the children constructed banks from milk cartons to collect their tokens.

On the third and fourth days, the teacher and class generated a menu of rewards. The children proposed material rewards, including stickers, stars, pencils, erasers, and small toys, plus activities and social rewards, such as playing board games, doing puzzles, computer time, listening to music, drawing, and painting. Of all the social rewards, having lunch with the teacher was the most popular. The teacher made a laminated poster listing the children's reward choices and the number of tokens needed for each reward.

On the fifth day, the teacher began depositing the earned tokens in each student's bank at three designated times per day. The banks were stored on a high shelf in the front of the classroom during instructional time. At the end of the day, children could choose to spend their tokens for rewards on the menu or to save their tokens for higher priced rewards. (Lunch with the teacher was a high-priced reward that was limited to 2 days per week, to allow the teacher some respite.) As part of her math instruction, the teacher taught the children how to count their tokens and to exchange small denominations for higher denominations.

The intervention focused mainly on increasing on-task behavior and reducing disruptive behavior in class. The teacher also incorporated social skills training and friendship issues into class discussions. Because Tyrone's and Lance's mothers reported many problems on the CBCL, the school psychologist encouraged them to seek help in behavioral management and parenting skills. Tyrone's mother began counseling at a CMHC, but Lance's mother declined to seek help.

Teacher Reports at Time 2

Six months after initiation of the classroom token economy (Time 2), the teacher again completed a TRF for each of the three boys. All three boys had improved in adaptive functioning, as indicated by TRF scores in the normal range. As shown in Figure 7.5, Tyrone and Gerald also showed marked reductions in problem behavior, obtaining normal range

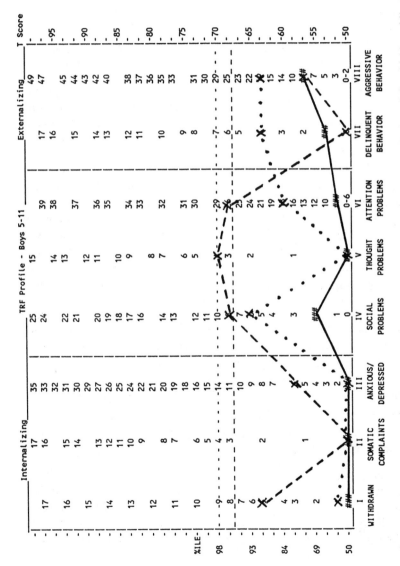

Figure 7.5. Time 2 TRF problem profiles for Tyrone (solid line), Lance (broken line), and Gerald (dotted line).

scores on all TRF problem scales. Tyrone's total problem raw score dropped 66 points from Time 1 to Time 2, demonstrating a very positive response to the school interventions. Gerald's total problem score dropped 29 points, although Gerald still scored above the 90th percentile for Social Problems. Lance showed little reduction in his Social Problems, Thought Problems, Attention Problems, or total problem scores.

The school psychologist used the DOF at Time 2 to rate the three boys' behavior in the classroom. The boys were now on-task 55% of the time, compared to 35% at Time 1. Tyrone improved the most, achieving 75% on-task behavior, whereas Lance improved the least, at 40%. Gerald was on-task 50% of the time. Tyrone and Gerald also improved on the DOF Externalizing and Hyperactive scales, with scores dropping into the normal range.

Summary of Tyrone, Lance, and Gerald

Tyrone, Lance, and Gerald illustrate the use of the TRF, DOF, and CBCL for planning and evaluating a group intervention. The Time 1 TRFs obtained from their first-grade teacher revealed severe problems in adaptive functioning and school behavior. DOFs completed by the school psychologist corroborated the teacher's reports, revealing low on-task scores and high scores for externalizing behavior and hyperactivity. CBCLs also produced high scores for attention problems for all three boys, as well as high scores for social problems and aggressive behavior for two boys.

The empirically based measures documented the need for a school-focused intervention, as well as mental health services for Tyrone and Lance. Their cognitive and achievement test scores indicated that Tyrone and Gerald's learning problems could not be attributed to low ability or learning disabilities. However, Lance's low scores on language and reading tests suggested needs for additional help in these areas. Because all three boys showed social and attention problems, as did some of their classmates, the teacher and school psychologist opted for a classwide token economy program, which the teacher could incorporate into her main mission of educating her pupils. The pupils became enthusiastic about earning rewards for improving their school behavior.

Time 2 TRFs indicated that Tyrone's and Gerald's behavior improved enough to reach the normal range on all problem scales. All three boys also showed improvement in TRF adaptive functioning and DOF on-task scores, indicating positive effects of the token economy. Lance, however, showed no improvement on the TRF Social Problems and Attention Problems scales, suggesting a need for more intensive interventions. Because Lance had obtained below-average scores on language and achievement tests at Time 1, he was referred for additional assessment to determine whether special education services were warranted. Lance's mother also reported family stresses leading to divorce that probably contributed to his problems, but she declined professional help for these problems.

Comparisons of the Time 1 and Time 2 TRFs indicated that Tyrone improved the most. A Time 2 CBCL completed by his mother indicated a 32-point drop in his total problem score, plus normal range scores on all syndrome scales. Tyrone's mother was the only one to seek professional help for behavior management. Gerald's mother had reported only social problems and some attention problems on the Time 1 CBCL, suggesting that his problems were confined to poor peer interactions and other problems in the school setting. Gerald's and Lance's mothers failed to complete Time 2 CBCLs.

In conclusion, the empirically based assessment indicated that the token economy was most effective in changing the behaviors on which it was specifically targeted, especially disruptive and on-task behavior. The combination of the token economy and professional help from the CMHC led to substantial improvements in home and school behavior for Tyrone. The school intervention alone led to better school behavior for Gerald, but less improvement for Lance, who showed language deficits and whose mother did not seek help for home-based problems.

SUMMARY

This chapter illustrated applications of empirically based assessment to special needs, including placement decisions for a retarded boy and an intervention for three boys that involved a token economy for their entire class. Even though Michael was known to be mentally retarded and to display very deviant behavior and thought problems, the empirically based procedures were useful for documenting the degree to which his behavior was deviant in particular areas, as reported by multiple informants. These included his mother who saw him at home, a child care worker who saw him in a residential treatment center, teachers who saw him in the center's school, and a foster parent who saw him in a therapeutic foster home. The empirically based measures were used to document stabilities and changes in his behavior in relation to different environments, the interventions that he received, and his increasing age. The findings were used in deciding on changes in placements, such as a possible return to his home and to mainstream or special education in a public school.

The similar TRF profiles found for Tyrone, Lance, and Gerald led to a token economy to improve their on-task behavior and to reduce the disruptive behavior that they had in common with each other and with several classmates. The TRFs provided baseline measures that documented the degree to which the boys' behavior was deviant and identified the specific areas of deviance to be targeted for change. The CBCLs completed by the boys' mothers yielded high Attention Problems scores that were consistent with their TRF scores. However, the boys differed more on other CBCL scales and in family factors that might affect their behavior.

Six months after the token economy began, the classroom learning atmosphere had improved, and outcome TRFs revealed marked improvements for Tyrone and Gerald. Less improvement was found for Lance, whose language deficits and family problems may have limited the efficacy of the classroom intervention. Thus, empirically based assessment initially indicated the desirability of a group intervention and then documented differences in outcomes among children who received the intervention.

8

ESSENTIAL FEATURES OF EMPIRICALLY BASED ASSESSMENT

In this chapter, we present essential features of the approach that was detailed in the preceding chapters. These features can be summarized as follows:

1. Empirically based assessment taps the ways in which children are seen by multiple informants, such as parents, teachers, practitioners, observers, and the children themselves.

2. Because empirically based assessment does not presuppose a particular theory about the nature or course of maladaptive behavior, it is compatible with most other approaches to children's problems and competencies.

3. Empirically based assessment adheres to psychometric guidelines, such as the following:

   a. Procedures are standardized.

   b. Multiple items are used to sample each aspect of functioning.

   c. Items are aggregated to provide quantitative scales for measuring each aspect of functioning.

   d. Scales are normed to facilitate comparisons of individual children with relevant reference groups of peers.

   e. For aspects of functioning that are related to development, normative reference groups are formed according to indices of development, such as age.

   f. To ensure psychometric soundness, the assessment procedures are tested for reliability and validity.

4. Because children's functioning may vary from one context to another, multiple sources and types of assessment data are needed, such as the following:

    a. Parent reports

    b. Teacher reports

    c. Cognitive assessment

    d. Physical assessment

    e. Direct assessment of the child, including self-reports, observations, and interviews

5. Procedures are available to help practitioners systematically compare reports by different informants about the same child.

6. The initial assessment procedures can be repeated periodically to measure changes and outcomes.

The empirically based procedures are compatible with other commonly used assessment procedures, including cognitive and achievement tests, family assessment, personality tests, developmental history interviews, behavioral assessment, medical examinations, and play sessions. They can be added to the practitioner's customary procedures with little cost or effort, while contributing data not likely to be obtained by other methods.

Empirically based assessment aims to sharpen, standardize, and document descriptions of children's functioning as seen by different informants. The quantification of descriptive data enables practitioners to determine the degree of deviance indicated by each informant's reports and to measure change from one occasion to another, such as from pre- to post-intervention. The empirically based data can contribute directly to case formulations, the choice of interventions, and the evaluation of outcomes. As outlined in Chapter 3, a growing body of research is documenting the differential nature and correlates of the empirically based syndromes. Numerous studies have also demonstrated the applicability of the empirically based procedures to many kinds of behavioral, emotional, and medical conditions, types of interventions, and outcome evaluations. (Brown & Achenbach, 1996, provide references to over 1,700 published reports grouped according to some 300 topics.) To help readers locate particular applications of empirically based assessment, Table 8.1 lists our case illustrations by number, pages, name, age, reason for assessment, initial assessment procedures, diagnosis, interventions, and subsequent assessments.

TABLE 8.1 Summary of Case Illustrations

Case No.	Pages	Name	Age	Reason for Assessment	Assessment Procedures[a]	DSM-IV Diagnosis	Interventions[b]	Outcome Assessment[a]
1	2–13, 26–39	Kyle	12 15	Noncompliant, easily, distracted, fighting	CBCL TRF YSR SCICA Parent interview Physical exam WISC-III Achievement tests	CD	Behavior modification Social skills program Cognitive-behavioral therapy Family therapy Parent training Special education	CBCL TRF YSR Achievement tests Achievement tests
2	41–42, 110–128	Lonnie	7 8	Won't stay in seat, can't focus on work, disruptive, hyperactive learning problems	CBCL TRF DOF Parent interview Teacher interview Conners Scales SCICA WISC-III Gordon Diagnostic System Physical exam	ADHD	Ritalin Parent training Classroom accommodations Behavior modification Social skills program	Conners Scales CBCL TRF
3	128–144	Natalie	10 13	Extreme emotional reactions, crying, dependence, poor school work	CBCL TRF SCICA Parent interview WISC-III Hearing test Physical exam	Dysthymia	Math instruction Classroom accommodations Behavioral incentives Family therapy Special education Social skills program	CBCL TRF YSR Achievement tests

TABLE 8.1 (Continued)

Case No.	Pages	Name	Age	Reason for Assessment	Assessment Procedures[a]	DSM-IV Diagnosis	Interventions[b]	Outcome Assessment[a]
4	155-166	Julie	10 14 15	Shoplifting, staying out late, sexual promiscuity	CBCL TRF YSR SCICA Parent interview WISC-III Physical exam	CD	Court diversion program Psychotherapy Community service	CBCL TRF YSR
5	168-177	Michael	9 12	Violent behavior, strange ideas and behavior	CBCL TRF Parent interview WJPB-R	Mental retardation CD	Residential placement Haldol Special education	CBCL TRF YSR SSRS CTAB WJPB-R
6	177-185	Tyrone Lance Gerald	6 6 6	Conduct problems, poor school work, group intervention	CBCL TRF DOF Teacher interview McCarthy Scales Achievement tests		Token economy in school Parent counseling for Tyrone	CBCL TRF DOF

a. Unfamiliar acronyms can be found in the List of Acronyms at the front of this book.
b. Note that the interventions were not necessarily the only ones or the best ones. Other practitioners might choose different interventions under similar conditions.

ASSESSMENT QUESTIONS

Empirically based assessment can help practitioners answer many kinds of questions that arise in contexts such as managed care, schools, mental health services, residential treatment, child custody and placement, child abuse, and delinquency. Empirically based assessment is also applicable to behavioral/emotional functioning associated with illness, physical disabilities, and mental retardation. As illustrated in the previous chapters, each case may pose a variety of questions. For example, a particular case may simultaneously raise questions about child custody, placement, abuse, and delinquency adjudication. Furthermore, a particular child may be retarded, ill, and have a physical disability. Because it is seldom possible to understand a child's needs solely in terms of a single assessment question, our empirically based procedures can be integrated with other procedures to address multiple questions about children's functioning. The specific procedures, sequences of assessment, and integrations of findings can be tailored to the questions that need to be answered, as summarized in the following sections.

Long-Term Versus Short-Term Problems

A question that arises in many cases is whether a child's behavioral and emotional problems reflect persistent long-term patterns or whether they reflect short-term, developmentally specific, reactive, or situational problems. This question is especially important for practitioners who serve organizations that have long-term responsibilities for children, such as schools and HMOs. Such organizations need to tailor services according to whether problems are acute or chronic. For example, based on the research that was reviewed in Chapter 3 and the specifics of their cases, the adolescent-onset delinquent behavior manifested by Julie (Case 4) was more likely to be specific to a particular developmental period and to particular environmental conditions than was the aggressive behavior manifested by Kyle (Case 1). Interventions for Julie could therefore concentrate on helping her develop more mature ways of coping with peer and family issues. If such interventions could capitalize on Julie's remorse for shoplifting, her motivation to change, and her attachment to her adoptive parents, the risk for persistent behavior problems appeared to be relatively low.

Kyle, on the other hand, showed a pattern of recurring aggressive behavior across developmental periods, situations, and changes in peer groups. Interventions were effective in changing specific problem behaviors and in helping Kyle progress in academic and vocational skills. However, a realistic long-term management plan would include continual monitoring and intervention to maintain control over his aggressive behavior.

Differences in the Implications of Particular Problems

Other questions concern possible differences in the implications of particular kinds of problems when they occur in boys versus girls and within different overall patterns of functioning. For example, both Lonnie (Case 2) and Natalie (Case 3) manifested attention problems, social problems, and poor school performance. However, empirically based assessment procedures revealed important differences between them. Lonnie's CBCL, TRF, and DOF yielded Attention Problems and Hyperactivity scores that were well up in the clinical range. His other problems varied more from one context to another. Interventions that included stimulant medication, behavior modification, and parent training were followed by substantial reductions in problem behavior.

Natalie's scores on the Attention Problems syndrome varied more between home and school than did Lonnie's. However, her profiles yielded more consistently deviant scores on the Social Problems syndrome and more evidence for affective problems than did Lonnie's. Ten *DSM-IV* symptoms of ADHD were reported for Natalie, but five were from the ADHD Inattention Type and five were from the Hyperactivity-Impulsivity Type. She thus fell short of the six of one or both types required for a diagnosis for ADHD. Attention problems certainly impaired Natalie's school performance, but her social and affective problems were also major sources of impairment.

Individual Versus Group Interventions

Interventions for behavioral and emotional problems are usually applied to individuals who are evaluated and treated one by one. In some cases, however, group interventions may be more therapeutically effective, as well as being more cost effective. Empirically based assessment can facilitate choices between individual and group interventions by helping practitioners identify children whose profile patterns are similar enough to be candidates for group interventions. When children with similar profiles are identified in settings where group interventions are feasible, the profiles can guide the interventions. Following an intervention, the empirically based procedures can be readministered to evaluate outcomes by comparing the scale scores obtained by each child before and after the intervention.

As an example, Tyrone, Lance, and Gerald (Case 6) obtained rather similar profiles of scores on TRFs completed by their first-grade teacher. Because of their mothers' concern that they not be singled out and because other children in the class manifested similar disruptive behavior, the school psychologist and teacher designed a token economy for the class. TRFs completed after the intervention yielded scores in the normal range on all scales for Tyrone and Gerald. Lance's behavior showed less consistent improvement, perhaps owing to his language deficits and more significant home-based problems for which his mother declined to seek help.

In addition to schools, other settings that serve groups of children can use empirically based assessment to distinguish between children whose patterns are idiosyncratic enough to warrant individual interventions and those whose patterns are similar enough to warrant group interventions. Examples of such settings include HMOs, residential treatment centers, psychiatric hospitals, and group homes.

Questions About Placements

Questions about alternative placements must be addressed when children's adaptive functioning or home situations are very poor. Michael (Case 5) was placed in a residential treatment center at age 9 when his behavior became too dangerous to be controlled at home, even with home-based services from a state agency. To deal with the problems resulting from his mental retardation, aggression, intermittent psychotic processes, and very poor academic and social skills, Michael remained in a group home operated by the residential center for 2 years. At age 11, he was moved to a therapeutic foster home operated by the residential center, but he continued to attend the center's school.

Because Michael was nearing the upper age limit of the residential center's services and because of the state's commitment to mainstreaming, it was necessary to determine whether Michael could be returned to his mother's home and a public school. CBCLs and TRFs obtained at his initial residential placement and periodically thereafter indicated definite improvement in several areas, including a decrease in aggression. However, according to multiple informants, Michael's scores on the Aggressive Behavior syndrome increased again by age 12, while his scores on the Social Problems and Thought Problems syndromes remained relatively high over the 3-year period. The overall picture of good responses to therapeutic environments, but persistently high levels of disturbed thinking and a resurgence of aggressive behavior argued for continued placement in settings geared to his special needs.

PATTERNS OF PROBLEMS

Procedures for assessing behavioral and emotional problems serve as tools for answering particular questions. In addition, the patterns of problems identified by the empirically based syndromes provide a conceptual framework for thinking about the similarities and differences among troubled children and their respective needs. The numerous correlates found for the syndromes (reviewed in Chapter 3) flesh out the conceptual framework in ways that can help us understand more about the patterns that are manifested by particular children. The following sections highlight some of the patterns that were illustrated by the cases presented in Chapters 5 through 7.

Affective Problems

The cross-informant syndrome designated as Anxious/Depressed reflects co-occurring problems of anxiety and depression that are often assigned to separate diagnostic categories. Although anxiety and depression may certainly occur separately, the Anxious/Depressed syndrome is consistent with the concept of negative affectivity, which is a general disposition to experience discomfort across diverse situations that are not stressful for most people (Watson & Clark, 1984). The Anxious/Depressed syndrome is also consistent with evidence that the same genetic factors influence anxiety and depressive disorders (Kendler et al., 1995).

Problems from the Anxious/Depressed syndrome were reported for several of our cases. However, they were most central for Natalie (Case 3), who obtained high scores on the TRF and SCICA Anxious/Depressed syndromes. Following school-based interventions to improve her academic and social skills, Natalie's TRF Anxious/Depressed scores indicated a considerable reduction in problems, but they remained in the clinical range. Natalie's Attention Problems score dropped from the borderline clinical range on her initial TRF to well within the normal range on outcome TRFs, although it was in the borderline range on her outcome CBCL. Her school behavior had thus improved considerably, but the outcome ratings indicated that she was liable to remain vulnerable to problems of the Anxious/Depressed and Attention Problems syndromes.

Attention Problems

As reviewed in Chapter 3, scores on the empirically based Attention Problems syndrome have yielded heritabilities of .47 to .79 and substantial developmental continuity. The Attention Problems syndrome is also significantly associated with *DSM-III* and *DSM-III-R* diagnoses of ADHD.

Unlike *DSM-III* and *DSM III-R, DSM-IV* divides ADHD into the three categories of Inattentive Type, Hyperactive-Impulsive Type, and Combined Type. To our knowledge, findings have not yet been published on relations between the Attention Problems syndrome and *DSM-IV* diagnoses of ADHD, and few findings have been published on relations between *DSM-IV* and previous *DSM* criteria for ADHD. However, in a study that applied both *DSM-III-R* and *DSM-IV* criteria to teachers' reports on a large general population sample, the *DSM-IV* criteria were found to classify 85% more girls and 50% more boys as having ADHD than the *DSM-III-R* criteria (Wolraich, Hannah, Pinnock, Baumgaertel, & Brown, 1996). These big increases—to a prevalence of 6.1% for girls and 16.2% for boys— raise questions about whether the *DSM-IV* criteria reflect the same diagnostic entity as the *DSM-III-R* criteria.

Linking the Attention Problems Syndrome to the DSM-IV *Types.* To cope with changes from one edition of *DSM* to another, practitioners may wish to link findings on the empirically based syndromes with whatever *DSM* criteria are currently in use. It may therefore be helpful to distinguish between subsets of items from our Attention Problems syndrome that primarily reflect inattention versus hyperactivity-impulsivity. To identify subsets of co-occurring items within the Attention Problems syndrome, we factor analyzed the 20 items of the TRF Attention Problems scale, as scored for the large clinical samples from which the TRF syndrome scales were derived (Achenbach, 1991c). The 20 items of the TRF Attention Problems scale tap more diverse problems than are tapped by the 11 items

TABLE 8.2   Inattention and Hyperactivity-Impulsivity Items of the TRF Attention Problems Scale

Inattention Items	Hyperactivity-Impulsivity Items	Items Associated With Both Subscales
4. Fails to finish things	1. Acts too young for age	8. Can't concentrate
13. Confused	2. Hums, makes odd	22. Difficulty following
17. Daydreams	noises	directions
49. Difficulty learning	10. Can't sit still	72. Messy work
60. Apathetic	15. Fidgets	78. Easily distracted
61. Poor schoolwork	41. Impulsive	
62. Clumsy	45. Nervous	
80. Stares blankly		
92. Underachieving		
100. Fails to carry out assigned tasks		

NOTE: The subsets of items were identified by factor analyzing TRFs for clinically referred children. Items are designated by the numbers they bear on the TRF and summaries of their content.

of the CBCL and 9 items of the YSR Attention Problem scales. The more numerous and diverse items of the TRF Attention Problems scale provide a more differentiated basis for constructing subscales than do the CBCL and YSR Attention Problems scales.

Table 8.2 lists two subsets of co-occurring items that were identified by factor analyzing the TRF Attention Problems scale. One subset consists primarily of items indicative of inattention, whereas the second subset consists primarily of items indicative of hyperactivity-impulsivity. In addition, the four items in the right-hand column of Table 8.2 were strongly associated with both subsets. In other words, these four items reflect characteristics that the two subsets of items have in common.

If a child's score on the entire TRF Attention Problems scale does not reach the borderline clinical range, the practitioner can compute separate scores for the subsets of items in Table 8.2. To compute the child's score for the inattention items, simply sum the child's scores on the items in the left column of Table 8.2. Similarly, to compute the child's score on the subset of hyperactivity-impulsivity items, sum the child's scores on the items in the middle column of Table 8.2. Because the four items in the right-hand column are strongly associated with both subsets of items, the next step is to add the scores obtained by the child on these four items to the sum for the inattention items and also to the sum for the hyperactivity-impulsivity items.

As a rule of thumb, practitioners can consider scores that are at or above the 95th percentile of the TRF normative sample for either subset of items to indicate deviance. Based on the TRF national norms (Achenbach, 1991c), the 95th percentile scores for each gender/age group are as follows:

1. For the sum of the inattention items, plus the four additional items: Boys 5 to 11 years old = 19; boys 12 to 18 = 21; girls 5 to 11 = 16; girls 12 to 18 = 15.
2. For the sum of the hyperactive-impulsive items, plus the four additional items: Boys 5 to 11 years old = 15; boys 12 to 18 = 14; girls 5 to 11 = 10; girls 12 to 18 = 9.

Differences between children who scored high on the Attention Problems syndrome were illustrated by Lonnie (Case 2) and Natalie (Case 3). Based on the CBCL, TRF, SCICA, and DOF, Lonnie manifested numerous problems of inattention and hyperactivity-impulsivity, which met criteria for a *DSM-IV* diagnosis of ADHD-Combined Type. Natalie's scores on the Attention Problems syndrome reached the clinical range on the CBCL and the borderline clinical range on the TRF, but she did not meet criteria for any of the three *DSM-IV* types of ADHD. However, her scores did reach the 95th percentile for 5- to 11-year-old girls on both subsets of items shown in Table 8.2. Although Natalie's attentional problems were less conspicuous than Lonnie's and did not meet *DSM-IV* criteria for ADHD, they did impair her functioning and needed to be considered in helping her.

Conduct Problems

The term *conduct problems* refers both to aggressive behavior and to nonaggressive delinquent behavior that violates social mores. Some children meet criteria for *DSM-IV* diagnoses of CD by manifesting only aggressive behavior, such as bullying, fighting, and cruelty. Other children meet criteria for CD by manifesting only nonaggressive delinquent behavior, such as lying, stealing, and truancy. Still others meet criteria for CD by manifesting both kinds of behavior.

Data on many samples of children assessed with numerous instruments have yielded a distinction between patterns of mainly aggressive versus mainly delinquent behavior (Achenbach, 1992a, and Quay, 1986, have provided reviews). Evidence reviewed in Chapter 3 indicates that the aggressive pattern is more persistent across long developmental periods and has stronger biological correlates than the delinquent pattern. Most children manifest at least some aggressive and delinquent behavior at certain points in their lives, but children who manifest a primarily aggressive pattern differ in important ways from those who manifest a primarily delinquent pattern. As illustrated by Kyle (Case 1) and Julie (Case 4), the contingencies affecting the aggressive versus delinquent patterns, their developmental course, and the therapeutic considerations may differ in important ways that are obscured by viewing conduct problems as a single category.

ASSESSING COMPETENCE

Although most referrals are prompted by concern about children's problems, their competencies are equally important. Some children's problems may primarily involve a lack of needed competencies. The best way to help such children may be to teach them adaptive skills. In other cases, a child may already have competencies that can help in coping with disabilities or stressors. In all cases, competencies should be assessed in order to provide a clear picture of a child's strengths and the areas in which competencies need to be strengthened, as well as areas in which problems need to be reduced.

Cognitive competencies can be assessed with standardized tests of ability and achievement but assessment of social competence is in an earlier stage of development. Our approach to assessing competence uses informants' reports of children's constructive activities, social relationships, and achievements to compare each child with what is reported for normative samples of peers. Our competence items have been shown to discriminate significantly between referred and nonreferred children and to add discriminative power to the assessment of problems (Achenbach, 1991b, 1991c, 1991d). Our procedures also assess different aspects of competence than are assessed by instruments such as the SSRS (Gresham & Elliott, 1990) and the CTAB (Adams, 1984). The complementary contributions of the SSRS, CTAB, and our procedures in the assessment of a mentally retarded child were illustrated in the case of Michael (Case 5).

SPECIAL ISSUES

Here we address some special issues that span multiple procedures. Issues arising in the use of particular instruments are detailed in the manuals for those instruments (Achenbach, 1991b, 1991c, 1991d, 1992b, 1993; McConaughy & Achenbach, 1994b).

Flexibility in Applying
Empirically Based Assessment

The empirically based procedures are designed to be flexibly adapted to the specific assessment needs and realities of each case. It is desirable to obtain standardized assessment data representing all five axes, but failure to do so does not negate the value of whichever procedures are feasible in a particular case. For example, if it is impractical to obtain teacher ratings or school observations for a child who attends school, it is nevertheless desirable to obtain parent and interviewer ratings, as well as medical and cognitive assessments. If medical and cognitive data are already available from relatively recent assessments, then these would not need to be repeated. For children who do not live with their parents, CBCLs can be completed by parent surrogates, such as relatives, foster parents, and child care workers, as illustrated in the assessment of Julie and Michael (Cases 4 and 5).

Comparisons between empirically based assessment procedures are most effective when the forms completed by different informants are done within about a month of each other. Comparisons across longer intervals can also be useful. However, the longer the interval between reports, the bigger the discrepancies may become because of changes in the child.

In addition to flexibility in applying and interpreting our procedures, flexibility is also needed in choosing other procedures to accompany them. As our case illustrations show, numerous procedures are compatible with ours, such as the WISC-III (Wechsler, 1991), WJPB-R (Woodcock & Johnson; 1989), GDS (Gordon, 1988), SSRS (Gresham & Elliott, 1990), CTAB (Adams, 1984), and CPRS/CTRS (Conners (1990). Other procedures, such as personality tests, behavioral assessment, and family assessment, may also be relevant in particular cases. Each procedure should be judged according to whether it adds reliable, valid, and cost-effective information on which to base important decisions.

Monitoring Changes and Outcomes

We have stressed the importance of repeated assessments to monitor changes in behavior over time, to evaluate the effects of interventions, and to provide a basis for continued planning. The empirically based procedures tap characteristics that may not show much change over very brief periods. It is therefore important to provide enough time between repeated assessments of a child for meaningful changes to occur, for the changes to become reasonably stable, and for informants to become aware of the changes. Accordingly, at least 2 months should typically be allowed between administrations of the CBCL, TRF, and YSR.

Readministration of the CBCL, TRF, and YSR at intervals as short as 2 months may be suitable for evaluating changes during an intervention in order to determine whether the intervention should be modified. However, for evaluating outcomes, a longer interval, such as 6 months, may be more appropriate to ensure that changes have become stable and to avoid placebo effects that may be associated with the onset of interventions. For greater certainty in evaluating the stability of outcomes, it is helpful to repeat the outcome assessments at additional intervals, such as 12 months and 18 months after the initial assessment.

To assess changes in groups of children, such as those participating in the evaluation of a particular intervention, it is important to use an interval between pre- and post-intervention assessments that is as uniform as possible for all participants. For example, if the intervention is of variable durations of up to 4 months, outcome assessments should be scheduled to be administered at a uniform interval greater than 4 months after the pre-intervention assessment, such as 6 months. Otherwise, if the reassessment intervals vary much, differences in the reassessment intervals could be confounded with effects of the intervention.

The CBCL/4-18 and YSR instruct respondents to base ratings on a 6-month period. This instruction can be changed to specify a shorter interval if needed. If a reassessment is scheduled for less than 6 months after the initial assessment, respondents should be instructed to base their initial ratings on an interval of the same length as is used for the reassessment. For example, if children are to be reassessed after an interval of 3 months, respondents should be instructed to use a 3-month basis for their initial ratings, as well as for each subsequent set of ratings. Because ratings of the TRF problem items are based on a 2-month interval, it would seldom be necessary to shorten this interval.

The SCICA and DOF ratings are based on a specific observational period. Consequently, they can be used to reassess children over any intervals, with no change in procedure. The DOF, in particular, can be used to reassess behavior over brief intervals to measure short-term changes in response to specific environmental manipulations or psychotropic drugs. However, to obtain representative samples of behavior even over brief intervals, it is desirable to average DOF scores over three or more 10-minute observation periods.

Crossing Between Age Periods

Reassessments sometimes span age periods that are scored on different instruments or in relation to norms for different age ranges, as discussed in the following sections.

Transitions From CBCL/2-3 to CBCL/4-18. If children who are initially assessed with the CBCL/2-3 are reassessed at age 4, it may be preferable to repeat the CBCL/2-3, rather than using the CBCL/4-18. By using the same instrument at both assessments, the practitioner can compare the child's scores on precisely the same items and scales. However, if reassessments are to be done after about the age of $4\frac{1}{2}$, it would usually be preferable to use the CBCL/4-18, because its items and norms become increasingly appropriate as children grow older. If individual children are assessed with the CBCL/2-3 and are subsequently reassessed with the CBCL/4-18, comparisons can be made in terms of T scores on the following scales, which show significant longitudinal correlations from age 3 to later ages (Achenbach, 1992b): Aggressive Behavior, Anxious/Depressed, Somatic Problems, Withdrawn, Internalizing, Externalizing, and total problems. When statistically comparing changes from CBCL/2-3 to CBCL/4-18 scores in different groups of children, such as those receiving different interventions, users can separately convert the CBCL/2-3 and CBCL/4-18 scores to standard scores within the entire sample being analyzed. The standard scores will provide a common metric across the different instruments.

Transitions From Child to Adolescent Norms. Across the ages for which the CBCL/4-18 and TRF are designed, the only change in the norms is from ages below 12 versus 12 to 18. Because the instruments remain the same across the entire age range, a child's raw item and scale scores can be compared across any interval. If the child is assessed before age 12 and is then reassessed after age 12, the child's T scores at each age can be used to determine how the child compares with agemates at each assessment. Thus, for example, a boy who obtained a raw score of 5 on the CBCL Delinquent Behavior scale would obtain a T score of 67 on the basis of norms for ages 4 to 11. However, a raw score of 5 on the CBCL Delinquent Behavior scale would obtain a T score of 63 on the basis of norms for ages 12 to 18. This is because scores on the Delinquent Behavior scale are higher for our normative samples of nonreferred adolescents than for pre-adolescents. As a result, a particular raw score, such as 5, ranks lower in the overall distribution of scores for adolescents than for pre-adolescents and therefore receives a lower T score for ages 12 to 18 than for ages 4 to 11.

Most of the scales do not show such large differences as the CBCL Delinquent Behavior scale between norms for adjoining age groups. However, the example of the Delinquent Behavior scale highlights differences that can arise between raw scores and T scores at different ages. For some kinds of problems, such as delinquent behavior, interventions that prevent increases in problems may effectively bring a child's functioning more into the normal range at ages when there is a general increase in such problems. Other kinds of problems, such as those on the CBCL Aggressive Behavior scale, may become less prevalent at ages 12 to 18 than 4 to 11. A boy whose raw scale score does not decline might therefore be more deviant relative to his peers at ages 12 to 18 than he was at ages 4 to 11. When evaluating changes in problems from one developmental period to another, it is thus important to consider both the absolute magnitude of problems, as indicated by raw scale scores, and the child's standing relative to peers of the same age range and gender, as indicated by T scores.

As Jacobson and Truax (1991) have pointed out, an important criterion for the clinical significance of intervention effects is whether the target problems decline from the clinical to the normal range. The clinical, borderline clinical, and normal ranges on the empirically based scales help practitioners judge the clinical significance of changes according to the Jacobson and Truax recommendation. Furthermore, the age-based norms for each gender provide practitioners with standards that take account of age changes in the prevalence of the problems scored on each scale, as illustrated for Kyle, Natalie, Julie, and Michael (Cases 1, 3, 4, and 5).

Transitions From Adolescence to Adulthood. For reassessments above age 18, the YABCL can be completed by parents and surrogates, while the YASR can be completed by the people who are being reassessed. As summarized in Chapter 3, several of the cross-informant syndromes scored from the CBCL/4-18 and YSR have substantial predictive correlations with analogous syndromes scored on the YABCL and YASR. These include the Aggressive Behavior, Anxious/Depressed, Delinquent Behavior, Somatic Complaints, and Withdrawn syndromes. Furthermore, substantial predictive correlations have been found from the adolescent Aggressive Behavior syndrome to the adult Shows Off syndrome scored on both the YABCL and YASR, and from the adolescent Attention Problems and Social Problems syndromes to their adult counterparts, which are scored only on the YABCL. The Internalizing, Externalizing, and total problem scales have also yielded substantial mean 3-year correlations ranging from .59 to .62 between adolescent CBCL/4-18 and YSR scores, on the one hand, and adult YABCL and YASR scores, on the other (Achenbach et al., 1995c).

There is thus considerable continuity between the adolescent and adult scales, despite changes in items to take account of developmental changes. For 18 year olds, practitioners may elect to use the adult instruments in cases where they appear to be more appropriate than the CBCL/4-18 and YSR, such as youths living away from their parents. Normed profiles for scoring the YABCL and YASR are scheduled for publication in 1997 (Achenbach, in press).

Special Populations

The syndrome scales of the CBCL, TRF, and YSR were derived from ratings of American children receiving mental health services or special education classes in diverse settings. The norms were constructed from ratings on national samples of American children who had not received mental health services or special education classes during the preceding year. Ethnic differences in item and scale scores have been minimal in analyses that controlled for socioeconomic status (Achenbach, 1991b, 1991c, 1991d, 1992b). The samples on which the DOF and SCICA were developed came from less diverse settings.

The original versions of the forms and syndromes are in English, but translations are available in some 50 languages, with findings having been published for many of these languages (Brown & Achenbach, 1996, provide references). Furthermore, statistical analyses of ratings for large clinical samples of Israeli and Dutch children have provided cross-cultural support for the syndrome structure derived from the American clinical samples (Auerbach & Lerner, 1991; DeGroot, Koot, & Verhulst, 1994, 1996). The growing body of translations and cross-cultural research can help practitioners use the empirically based assessment forms with children from many language backgrounds besides English.

To avoid the possible effects of mental retardation and physical disabilities on the assessment of behavioral and emotional problems, children with these conditions were not included in the clinical or normative samples employed in developing the empirically based assessment procedures. However, to facilitate adaptation to mainstream and other nonrestrictive settings, practitioners often need to know how the behavioral and emotional problems and competencies of children with disabilities compare to those of children who do not have disabilities. If a child with a disability is found to have competence or problem scores in the clinical range on particular scales, the practitioner can target these areas for intervention or for environmental accommodations. The empirically based procedures can also be readministered periodically to determine whether the child's problems and competencies are improving, remaining the same, or worsening.

Relations to Interventions

Empirically based assessment can be used with almost any form of intervention, both to identify problems and competencies that are to be targeted for change and to assess the effects of interventions. Because empirically based assessment is not restricted to disorders having a particular etiology nor to particular types of interventions, it can be used to choose among intervention options. Other kinds of assessment may be used with empirically based assessment at the option of the practitioner. Examples include behavioral assessment for use in behavioral interventions; family assessment when family systems approaches are being considered; medical assessment to evaluate prospects for medication; personality tests for psychodynamically oriented therapy; curriculum-based assessment for educational interventions; and assessment of parents to determine their workability for various interventions.

Our cases illustrated the use of empirically based assessment in conjunction with the following interventions: behavioral incentives (Case 3); behavior modification (Cases 1, 2); classroom accommodations (Cases 2, 3); cognitive-behavioral therapy (Case 1); community service (Case 4);

court diversion program (Case 4); family therapy (Cases 1, 3); Haldol (Case 5); math instruction (Case 3); parent counseling (Case 6); parent training (Case 1); psychotherapy (Case 4); residential placement (Case 5); Ritalin (Case 2); social skills training (Cases 1, 2, 3); special education (Cases 1, 3, 5); token economy (Case 6).

CURRENT STATUS AND
FUTURE DIRECTIONS

The cases presented in Chapters 5, 6, and 7 have illustrated essential features of empirically based assessment, which taps the ways in which children are seen by various informants. It does not presuppose particular theories of maladaptive behavior but adheres to psychometric guidelines for assessing children under a variety of conditions and for systematically comparing reports by multiple informants.

The assessment procedures are economical, easy to use, and compatible with most other procedures. They are designed to sharpen, standardize, and document descriptions of children's functioning as seen by different informants. The quantification of descriptive data enables practitioners to determine degrees of deviance and to measure changes in reported behavior. A growing body of research documents the nature and correlates of the empirically based syndromes and their applications in many contexts.

We illustrated applications to assessment questions regarding chronic versus acute problems (Cases 1, 4); differences in the implications of particular problems (Cases 2, 3); individual versus group interventions (Case 6); and choices of placements (Case 5). We also illustrated the assessment of competencies and particular patterns of problems, including affective problems (Case 3); attention problems (Cases 2, 3); and conduct problems (Cases 1, 4, 5).

Special issues were addressed, including flexibility in applying empirically based assessment; monitoring changes and outcomes; crossing between age periods; special populations; and relations to particular interventions.

Our empirically based approach is designed to advance the understanding and amelioration of psychopathology. Although we have focused mainly on ages 4 to 18, multiaxial empirically based assessment also includes preschool children and young adults. The instruments for assessing these age groups include the CBCL/2-3, the TCRF/2-5, and the YABCL and YASR for young adults. These instruments are products of research on the developmental course of problems and competencies. They have contributed to the identification of continuities in problem patterns across multiple developmental periods. The period between the ages of 18 and the mid-20s presents assessment challenges arising from the variety of developmental paths that may be followed and from the less clear standards for judging deviance than apply at earlier and later ages. The extensions of our approach to young adults can help to fill gaps between assessment procedures that are geared to children and adolescents and those that are geared to older adults.

The rating forms and scoring procedures illustrated in this book are components of a paradigm for conceptualizing psychopathology in terms of empirically derived syndromal constructs. This paradigm is generating research on many aspects of psychopathology in ways that facilitate communication across disciplines and viewpoints. The common descriptive language provided by the paradigm also facilitates the training of practitioners and applications of research findings by practitioners. With mental health services increasingly dominated by managed care, the empirically based paradigm offers concepts and procedures that can be shared by practitioners from diverse backgrounds who must now meet common standards of accountability.

REFERENCES

Abramowitz, A. J., & O'Leary, S. G. (1991). Behavioral interventions for the classroom: Implications for students with ADHD. *School Psychology Review, 20,* 220-234.

Achenbach, T. M. (1966). The classification of children's psychiatric symptoms: A factor-analytic study. *Psychological Monographs, 80*(No. 615).

Achenbach, T. M. (1991a). *Integrative guide for the 1991 CBCL/4-18, YSR, and TRF profiles.* Burlington: University of Vermont, Department of Psychiatry.

Achenbach, T. M. (1991b). *Manual for the Child Behavior Checklist/4-18 and 1991 Profile.* Burlington: University of Vermont, Department of Psychiatry.

Achenbach, T. M. (1991c). *Manual for the Teacher's Report Form and 1991 Profile.* Burlington: University of Vermont, Department of Psychiatry.

Achenbach, T. M. (1991d). *Manual for the Youth Self-Report and 1991 Profile.* Burlington: University of Vermont, Department of Psychiatry.

Achenbach, T. M. (1992a). Developmental psychopathology. In M. H. Bornstein & M. E. Lamb (Eds.), *Developmental psychology: An advanced textbook* (3rd ed.). Hillsdale, NJ: Lawrence Erlbaum.

Achenbach, T.M. (1992b). *Manual for the Child Behavior Checklist/2-3 and 1992 Profile.* Burlington: University of Vermont, Department of Psychiatry.

Achenbach, T. M. (1993). *Empirically based taxonomy: How to use syndromes and profile types derived from the CBCL/4-18, TRF, and YSR.* Burlington: University of Vermont, Department of Psychiatry.

Achenbach, T. M. (1995). *Teacher/Caregiver Report Form for Ages 2-5.* Burlington: University of Vermont, Department of Psychiatry.

Achenbach, T. M. (in press). *Manual for the Young Adult Behavior Checklist and Young Adult Self-Report.* Burlington: University of Vermont, Department of Psychiatry.

Achenbach, T. M., Conners, C. K., Quay, H. C., Verhulst, F. C., & Howell, C. T. (1989). Replication of empirically derived syndromes as a basis for taxonomy of child/adolescent psychopathology. *Journal of Abnormal Child Psychology, 17,* 299-323.

Achenbach, T. M., & Howell, C. T. (1993). Are American children's problems getting worse? A 13-year comparison. *Journal of the American Academy of Child and Adolescent Psychiatry, 32,* 1145-1154.

Achenbach, T. M., Howell, C. T., McConaughy, S. H., & Stanger, C. (1995a). Six-year predictors of problems in a national sample of children and youth: I. Cross-informant syndromes. *Journal of the American Academy of Child and Adolescent Psychiatry, 34,* 336-347.

Achenbach, T. M., Howell, C. T., McConaughy, S. H., & Stanger, C. (1995b). Six-year predictors of problems in a national sample of children and youth: II. Signs of disturbance. *Journal of the American Academy of Child and Adolescent Psychiatry, 34,* 488-498.

Achenbach, T. M., Howell, C. T., McConaughy, S. H., & Stanger, C. (1995c). Six-year predictors of problems in a national sample: III. Transitions to young adult syndromes. *Journal of the American Academy of Child and Adolescent Psychiatry, 34,* 658-669.

Achenbach, T. M., & McConaughy, S. H. (1987). *Empirically based assessment of child and adolescent psychopathology: Practical applications.* Newbury Park, CA: Sage.

Achenbach, T. M., McConaughy, S. H., & Howell, C. T. (1987). Child/adolescent behavioral and emotional problems: Implications of cross-informant correlations for situational specificity. *Psychological Bulletin, 101,* 213-232.

Adams, G. L. (1984). *Comprehensive test of adaptive behavior.* New York: Psychological Corporation.

American Psychiatric Association. (1980). *Diagnostic and statistical manual of mental disorders* (3rd ed.). Washington, DC: Author.

American Psychiatric Association. (1987). *Diagnostic and statistical manual of mental disorders* (3rd ed. rev.). Washington, DC: Author.

American Psychiatric Association. (1994). *Diagnostic and statistical manual of mental disorders* (4th ed.). Washington, DC: Author.

Angold, A., & Costello, E. J. (1991). Developing a developmental epidemiology. In D. Cicchetti & S. L. Toth (Eds.), *Rochester Symposium on Developmental Psychopathology: Volume 3. Models and integrations* (pp. 75-96). Rochester, NY: University of Rochester Press.

Arnold, J. (1996). *The Client Entry Program for the CBCL/4-18, YSR, & TRF.* Burlington: University of Vermont, Department of Psychiatry.

Arnold, J., & Jacobowitz, D. (1993). *The Cross-Informant Program for the CBCL/4-18, YSR, & TRF.* Burlington: University of Vermont, Department of Psychiatry.

Auerbach, J. G., & Lerner, Y. (1991). Syndromes derived from the Child Behavior Checklist for clinically referred Israeli boys aged 6-11. *Journal of Child Psychology and Psychiatry, 32,* 1017-1024.

Barkley, R. A. (1987). *Defiant children: A clinician's manual for parent training.* New York: Guilford.

Barkley, R. A. (1990). *Attention Deficit Hyperactivity Disorder: A handbook for diagnosis and treatment.* New York: Guilford.

Barkley, R. A., DuPaul, G. J., & McMurray, M. B. (1990). Comprehensive evaluation of Attention Deficit Disorder with and without hyperactivity as defined by research criteria. *Journal of Consulting and Clinical Psychology, 58,* 775-789.

Bergman, A. J., & Walker, E. (1995). The relationship between cognitive functions and behavioral deviance in children at risk for psychopathology. *Journal of Child Psychology and Psychiatry, 36,* 265-278.

Birmaher, B., Stanley, M., Greenhill, L., Twomey, J., Gavrilescu, A., & Rabinovich, H. (1990). Platelet imipramine binding in children and adolescents with impulsive behavior. *Journal of the American Academy of Child and Adolescent Psychiatry, 29,* 914-918.

Brown, J. S., & Achenbach, T. M. (1996). *Bibliography of published studies using the Child Behavior Checklist and related materials: 1996 edition.* Burlington: University of Vermont, Department of Psychiatry.

Brown, R. T., Kaslow, N. J., Doepke, K., Buchanan, I., Eckman, J., Baldwin, K., & Goonan, B. (1993). Psychosocial and family functioning in children with sickle cell syndrome and their mothers. *Journal of the American Academy of Child and Adolescent Psychiatry, 32,* 545-553.

Brown, S.-L. & van Praag, H. M. (1991). *The role of serotonin in psychiatric disorders.* New York: Brunner/Mazel.

Cantor, N., Smith, E. E., French, R. deS., & Mezzich, J. (1980). Psychiatric diagnosis as prototype categorization. *Journal of Abnormal Psychology, 89,* 181-193.

Caron, C., & Rutter, M. (1991). Co-morbidity in child psychopathology: Concepts, issues, and research strategies. *Journal of Child Psychology and Psychiatry, 32,* 1063-1080.

Chen, W. J., Faraone, S. V., Biederman, J., & Tsuang, M. T. (1994). Diagnostic accuracy of the Child Behavior Checklist scales for Attention-Deficit Hyperactivity Disorder: A receiver-operating characteristic analysis. *Journal of Consulting and Clinical Psychology, 62,* 1017-1025.

Conners, C. K. (1973). Rating scales for use in drug studies with children. In *Psychopharmacology Bulletin: Pharmacotherapy with children.* Washington, DC: Government Printing Office.

Conners, C. K. (1990). *Conners' Rating Scales Manual.* North Tonawanda, NY: Multi-Health Systems.

Conrad, M., & Hammen, C. (1989). Role of maternal depression in perceptions of child maladjustment. *Journal of Consulting and Clinical Psychology, 57,* 663-667.

Costello, A. J., Edelbrock, C., Dulcan, M. K., Kalas, R., & Klaric, S. H. (1984). *Report on the Diagnostic Interview Schedule for Children (DISC).* Pittsburgh, PA: University of Pittsburgh, Department of Psychiatry.

Cowley, G., & Ramo, J. C. (1993, July 26). The not-young and the restless. *Newsweek,* pp. 48-49.

Cunningham, S. J., McGrath, P. J., Ferguson, H. B., Humphreys, P., Dastous, J., Latter, J., Firestone, P., & Goodman, J. T. (1987). Personality and behavioral characteristics in pediatric migraine. *Headache, 27,* 16-20.

Dawson, M. M. (1995). Best practices in planning interventions for students with attention disorders. In A. Thomas & J. Grimes (Eds.), *Best practice in school psychology III.* Washington, DC: National Association of School Psychologists.

De Groot, A., Koot, H. M., & Verhulst, F. C. (1994). Cross-cultural generalizability of the CBCL cross-informant syndromes. *Psychological Assessment, 6,* 225-230.

De Groot, A., Koot, H. M., & Verhulst, F. C. (in press). Cross-cultural generalizability of the Youth Self-Report and Teacher's Report Form cross-informant syndromes. *Journal of Abnormal Child Psychology, 25.*

DuPaul, G. J., & Stoner, G. (1994). *ADHD in the schools: Assessment and intervention strategies.* New York: Guilford.

Edelbrock, C., & Costello, A. J. (1988). Convergence between statistically derived behavior problem syndromes and child psychiatric diagnoses. *Journal of Abnormal Child Psychology, 16,* 219-231.

Edelbrock, C., Costello, A. J., Dulcan, M. K., Kalas, R., & Conover, N. C. (1985). Age differences in the reliability of the psychiatric interview of the child. *Child Development, 56,* 265-275.

Edelbrock, C., Rende, R., Plomin, R., & Thompson, L. A. (1995). A twin study of effects on competence and problem behavior in childhood and early adolescence. *Journal of Child Psychology and Psychiatry, 36,* 775-785.

Ernst, M., Liebenauer, L. L., King, A. C., Fitzgerald, G. A., Cohen, R. M., & Zametkin, A. J. (1994). Reduced brain metabolism in hyperactive girls. *Journal of the American Academy of Child and Adolescent Psychiatry, 33,* 858-868.

Eron, L. D., & Huesmann, L. R. (1990). The stability of aggressive behavior—Even unto the third generaton. In M. Lewis & S. Miller (Eds.), *Handbook of developmental psychopathology.* New York: Plenum.

Faraone, S. V., Biederman, J., Keenan, K., & Tsuang, M. T. (1991). Separation of *DSM-III* attention deficit disorder and conduct disorder: Evidence from a family-genetic study of American child psychiatric patients. *Psychological Medicine, 21,* 109-121.

Finch, A. J., Lipovsky, J. A., & Casat, C. D. (1989). Anxiety and depression in children and adolescents: Negative affectivity or separate constructs? In P. C. Kendall & D. Watson (Eds.), *Anxiety and depresson: Distinctive and overlapping features.* New York: Academic Press.

Friedlander, S., Weiss, D. S., & Traylor, J. (1986). Assessing the influence of maternal depression on the validity of the Child Behavior Checklist. *Journal of Abnormal Child Psychology, 14,* 123-133.

Gabel, S., Stadler, J., Bjorn, J., Shindledecker, R., & Bowden, C. (1993). Dopamine-beta-hydroxylase in behaviorally disturbed youth. Relationship between teacher and parent ratings. *Biological Psychiatry, 34,* 434-442.

Ghodsian-Carpey, J., & Baker, L. A. (1987). Genetic and environmental influences on aggression in 4- to 7-year-old twins. *Aggressive Behavior, 13,* 173-186.

Gjone, H., Stevenson, J., & Sundet, J. M. (1996). Genetic influence on parent-reported attention-related problems in a Norwegian general population twin sample. *Journal of the American Academy of Child and Adolescent Psychology, 35,* 588-596.

Goldstein, A. P. (1988). *The Prepare Curriculum.* Champaign, IL: Research Press.

Goldstein, S. (1995). *Understanding and managing children's classroom behavior.* New York: John Wiley.

Gordon, M. (1988). *Gordon Diagnostic System.* DeWitt, NY: Gordon Systems, Inc.

Gould, M. S., Bird, H., & Jaramillo, B. S. (1993). Correspondence between statistically derived behavior problem syndromes and child psychiatric diagnoses in a community sample. *Journal of Abnormal Child Psychology, 21,* 287-313.

Gove, P. (Ed.). (1971). *Webster's third new international dictionary of the English language.* Springfield, MA: Merriam.

Goyette, C. H., Conners, C. K., & Ulrich, R. F. (1978). Normative data on revised Conners Parent and Teacher Rating Scales. *Journal of Abnormal Child Psychology, 6,* 221-236.

Granger, D. A., Weisz, J. R., & Kauneckis, D. (1994). Neuroendocrine reactivity, internalizing behavior problems, and control-related cognitions in clinic-referred children and adolescents. *Journal of Abnormal Psychology, 103,* 267-276.

Gray, J. A. (1982). *The neuropsychology of anxiety: An inquiry into the function of the septo-hippocampal system.* New York: Oxford University Press.

Gray, J. A. (1987a). Perspectives on anxiety and impulsivity: A commentary. *Journal of Research in Personality, 21,* 493-509.

Gray, J. A. (1987b). *The psychology of fear and stress.* New York: Cambridge University Press.

Gresham, F. M., & Elliott, S. N. (1990). *Social skills rating system.* Circle Pines, MN: American Guidance Service.

Hampton, J. A. (1993). Prototype models of concept representation. In I. Van Mechelen, J. Hampton, R. S. Michalski, & P. Theuns (Eds.), *Categories and concepts: Theoretical views and inductive data analysis.* London: Academic Press.

Hanna, G. L. (1995). Demographic and clinical features of obsessive-compulsive disorder in children and adolescents. *Journal of the American Academy of Child and Adolescent Psychiatry, 34,* 19-27.

Hanna, G. L., Yuwiler, A., & Coates, J. K. (1995). Whole blood serotonin and disruptive behaviors in juvenile obsessive-compulsive disorder. *Journal of the American Academy of Child and Adolescent Psychiatry, 34,* 28-35.

Hart, E. L., Lahey, B. B., Loeber, R., Applegate, B., & Frick, P. J. (1995). Developmental change in attention-deficit hyperactivity disorder in boys: A four-year longitudinal study. *Journal of Abnormal Child Psychology, 23,* 729-749.

Helzer, J. E., Spitznagel, E. L., & McEvoy, L. (1987). The predictive validity of lay DIS diagnoses in the general population: A comparison with physician examiners. *Archives of General Psychiatry, 44,* 1069-1077.

Henn, F. A., Bardwell, R., & Jenkins, R. L. (1980). Juvenile delinquents revisited. Adult criminal activity. *Archives of General Psychiatry, 37,* 1160-1163.

Hewitt, L. E., & Jenkins, R. L. (1946). *Fundamental patterns of maladjustment: The dynamics of their origin.* Springfield: State of Illinois.

Hodges, K. (1993). Structured interviews for assessing children. *Journal of Child Psychology and Psychiatry, 34,* 49-68.

Hodges, K., Kline, J., Stern, L., Cytryn, L., & McKnew, D. (1982). The development of a child assessment interview for research and clinical use. *Journal of Abnormal Child Psychology, 10,* 173-189.

Horowitz, L. M., Post, D. L., French, R. deS., Wallis, K. D., & Siegelman, E. Y. (1981). The prototype as a construct in abnormal psychology: 2. Clarifying disagreement in psychiatric judgments. *Journal of Abnormal Psychology, 90,* 575-585.

Horowitz, L. M., Wright, J. C., Lowenstein, E., & Parad, H. W. (1981). The prototype as a construct in abnormal psychology: 1. A method for deriving prototypes. *Journal of Abnormal Psychology, 90,* 568-574.

Hughes, J., & Baker, D. B. (1990). *The clinical child interview.* New York: Guilford.

Individuals With Disabilities Education Act. (1990). Public Law 101-476. 20 U.S.C 1401.

Irwin, E. C. (1983). The diagnostic and therapeutic use of pretend play. In C. Schaefer & K. O'Connor (Eds.), *Handbook of play therapy* (pp. 148-173). New York: John Wiley.

Jacobowitz, D. (1996). *Program manual for the Scanvert Program to convert scanned data to raw data format.* Burlington: University of Vermont, Department of Psychiatry.

Jacobson, N. S., & Truax, P. (1991). Clinical significance: A statistical approach to defining meaningful change in psychotherapy research. *Journal of Consulting and Clinical Psychology, 59,* 12-19.

Jenkins, R. L., & Boyer, A. (1968). Types of delinquent behavior and background factors. *International Journal of Social Psychiatry, 14,* 65-76.

Jensen, P. S., Roper, M., Fisher, P., Piacentini, J., Canino, G., Richters, J., Rubio-Stipec, M., Dulcan, M., Goodman, S., Davies, M., Rae, D., Shaffer, D., Bird, H., Lahey, B., & Schwab-Stone, M. (1995). Test-retest reliability of the Diagnostic Interview Schedule for Children (ver. 2.1): Parent, child, and combined algorithms. *Archives of General Psychiatry, 52,* 61-71.

Jensen, P. S., Traylor, J., Xenakis, S. N., & Davis, H. (1988). Child psychopathology rating scales and interrater agreement: I. Parents' gender and psychiatric status. *Journal of the American Academy of Child and Adolescent Psychiatry, 27,* 442-450.

Johnston, L. D., O'Malley, P. M., & Bachman, J. G. (1995). *National survey results on drug use from the monitoring the future study, 1975-1994* (Vol. 1). Rockville, MD: National Institute on Drug Abuse.

Kagan, J. (1994). *Galen's prophecy: Temperament in human nature.* New York: Basic Books.

Kaufman, A. S., & Kaufman, N. L. (1983). *Kaufman Assessment Battery for Children.* Circle Pines, MN: American Guidance Service.

Kazdin, A. (1987). Treatment of antisocial behavior in children: Current status and future directions. *Psychological Bulletin, 102,* 187-203.

Kazdin, A., Esveldt-Dawson, K., French, N., & Unis, A. (1987). Effects of parent management training and problem-solving skills training combined in treatment of antisocial child behavior. *Journal of the American Academy of Child and Adolescent Psychiatry, 26,* 416-424.

Kelley, M. L. (1990). *School-home notes: Promoting children's classroom success.* New York: Guilford.

Kendall, P. C., & Panichelli-Mindel, S. M. (1995). Cognitive-behavioral treatments. *Journal of Abnormal Child Psychology, 23,* 107-124.

Kendler, K. S., Neale, M. C., Kessler, R. C., Heath, A. C., & Eaves, L. J. (1992). Major depression and generalized anxiety disorder: Same genes, (partly) different environments? *Archives of General Psychiatry, 49,* 716-722.

Kendler, K. S., Walters, E. E., Neale, M. C., Kessler, R. C., Heath, A. C., & Eaves, L. J. (1995). The structure of the genetic and environmental risk factors for six major psychiatric disorders in women. *Archives of General Psychiatry, 52,* 374-383.

King, N. J., Ollendick, T. H., & Gullone, E. (1991). Negative affectivity in children and adolescents: Relations between anxiety and depression. *Clinical Psychology Review, 11,* 441-459.

King, R. A., Scahill, L., Vitulano, L. A., Schwab-Stone, M., Tercyak, K. P., & Riddle, M. A. (1995). Childhood trichotillomania: Clinical phenomenology, co-morbidity, and family genetics. *Journal of the American Academy of Child and Adolescent Psychiatry, 34,* 1451-1459.

Koot, H. M. (1993). *Problem behavior in Dutch preschoolers.* Rotterdam, The Netherlands: Erasmus University, Sophia Children's Hospital.

Koppitz, E. M. (1975). *The Bender Gestalt Test for young children* (Vol. 2). New York: Grune & Stratton.

Kovacs, M. (1981). Rating scales to assess depression in school-aged children. *Acta Paedopsychiatrica, 46,* 305-315.

Kovacs, M., Gatsonis, C., Paulauskas, S. L., & Richards, C. (1989). Depressive disorders in childhood. IV. A longitudinal study of comorbidity with the risk for anxiety disorders. *Archives of General Psychiatry, 46,* 776-782.

Kuepper, J. E. (1987). *Homework helpers: A guide for parents offering assistance.* Minneapolis, MN: Educational Media Corporation.

Lahey, B. B., Loeber, R., Stouthamer-Loeber, M., Christ, M. A. G., Green, S., Russo, M. F., Frick, P. J., & Dulcan, M. (1990). Comparison of *DSM-III* and *DSM-III-R* diagnoses for prepubertal children: Changes in prevalence and validity. *Journal of the American Academy of Child and Adolescent Psychiatry, 29,* 620-626.

Landau, S., & Moore, L. A. (1991). Social skills deficits in children with Attention-Deficit Hyperactivity Disorder. *School Psychology Review, 20,* 235-251.

Loeber, R., & Schmaling, K. B. (1985). Empirical evidence for overt and covert patterns of antisocial conduct problems: A meta-analysis. *Journal of Abnormal Child Psychology, 13,* 337-352.

Mannuzza, S., Klein, R. G., Bessler, A., Malloy, P., & LaPadula, M. (1993). Adult outcome of hyperactive boys: Educational achievement, occupational rank, and psychiatric status. *Archives of General Psychiatry, 50,* 565-576.

McBurnett, K., Lahey, B. B., & Pfiffner, L. J. (1993). Diagnosis of attention deficit disorders in *DSM-IV:* Scientific basis and implications for education. *Exceptional Children, 60,* 108-117.

McCarthy, D. (1972). *McCarthy Scales of Children's Abilities.* New York: Psychological Corporation.

McConaughy, S. H. (1996). The interview process. In M. Breen & C. Fiedler (Eds.), *Behavioral approach to the assessment of youth with emotional/behavioral disorders: A handbook for school-based practitioners* (pp. 181-223). Austin, TX: PRO-ED.

McConaughy, S. H., & Achenbach, T. M. (1994a). Co-morbidity of empirically based syndromes in matched general population and clinical samples. *Journal of Child Psychology and Psychiatry, 35,* 1141-1157.

McConaughy, S. H., & Achenbach, T. M. (1994b). *Manual for the Semistructured Clinical Interview for Children and Adolescents.* Burlington: University of Vermont, Department of Psychiatry.

McConaughy, S. H., Achenbach, T. M., & Gent, C. L. (1988). Multiaxial empirically based assessment: Parent, teacher, observational, cognitive, and personality correlates of Child Behavior Profiles for 6-11-year-old boys. *Journal of Abnormal Child Psychology, 16,* 485-509.

McGee, M. F., Feehan, M., Williams, S., & Anderson, J. (1992). *DSM-III* disorders from age 11 to age 15 years. *Journal of the American Academy of Child and Adolescent Psychiatry, 31,* 50-59.

McGinnis, E., & Goldstein, A. P. (1984). *Skillstreaming the elementary school child.* Champaign, IL: Research Press.

McGinnis, E., Goldstein, A. P., Sprafkin, R., Gershaw, J., & Klein, P. (1980). *Skillstreaming the adolescent.* Champaign, IL: Research Press.

Moffitt, T. E. (1993). "Life-course persistent" and "adolescence-limited" antisocial behavior: A developmental taxonomy. *Psychological Review, 100,* 674-701.

Nunnally, J. C., & Bernstein, I. H. (1994). *Psychometric theory.* New York: McGraw-Hill.

Quay, H. C. (1986). Classification. In H. C. Quay & J. S. Werry (Eds.), *Psychopathological disorders of childhood* (3rd ed., pp. 1-42). New York: John Wiley.

Quay, H. C. (1993). The psychobiology of undersocialized aggressive conduct disorder: A theoretical perspective. *Development and Psychopathology, 5,* 165-180.

Quay, H. C., & Peterson, D. R. (1982). *Revised Behavior Problem Checklist.* Coral Gables, FL: University of Miami, Department of Psychology.

Rey, J. M., & Morris-Yates, A. (1992). Diagnostic accuracy in adolescents of several depression rating scales extracted from a general purpose behavior checklist. *Journal of Affective Disorders, 26,* 7-16.

Reynolds, C. R., & Kamphaus, R. W. (1992). *Behavior Assessment System for Children (BASC).* Circle Pines, MN: American Guidance Service.

Reynolds, C. R., & Richmond, B. O. (1978). What I Think and Feel: A revised measure of children's manifest anxiety. *Journal of Abnormal Child Psychology, 6,* 271-280.

Richters, J. E. (1992). Depressed mothers as informants about their children: A critical review of the evidence for distortion. *Psychological Bulletin, 112,* 485-499.

Richters, J. E., & Pellegrini, D. (1989). Depressed mothers' judgments about their children: An examination of the depression-distortion hypothesis. *Child Development, 60,* 1068-1075.

Robins, L. N. (1985). Epidemiology: Reflections on testing the validity of psychiatric interviews. *Archives of General Psychiatry, 42,* 918-924.

Rosch, E. (1978). Principles of categorization. In E. Rosch & B. B. Lloyd (Eds.), *Cognition and categorization.* Hillsdale, NJ: Lawrence Erlbaum.

Rosch, E., & Mervis, C. B. (1975). Family resemblances: Studies in the internal structure of categories. *Cognitive Psychology, 7,* 573-605.

Routh, D. K., & Ernst, A. R. (1984). Somatization disorder in relatives of children and adolescents with functional abdominal pain. *Journal of Pediatric Psychology, 9,* 427-437.

Sawyer, M. G. (1990). *Childhood behavior problems: Discrepancies between reports from children, parents, and teachers.* Unpublished doctoral dissertation. University of Adelaide, Australia.

Scerbo, A. S., & Kolko, D. (1994). Salivary testosterone and cortisol in disruptive children: Relationship to aggressive, hyperactive, and internalizing behaviors. *Journal of the American Academy of Child and Adolescent Psychiatry, 33,* 1174-1184.

Schmitz, S., Fulker, D. W., & Mrazek, D. A. (1995). Problem behavior in early and middle childhood: An initial behavior genetic analysis. *Journal of Child Psychology and Psychiatry, 36,* 1443-1458.

Semel, E., Wiig, E. H., & Secord, W. (1987). *Clinical Evaluation of Language Fundamentals-Revised.* New York: Psychological Corporation.

Skiba, R., & Grizzle, K. (1991). The social maladjustment exclusion: Issues of definition and assessment. *School Psychology Review, 20,* 577-595.

Skiba, R., & Grizzle, K. (1992). Qualifications v. logic and data: Excluding conduct disorders from the SED definition. *School Psychology Review, 21,* 23-28.

Slenkovich, J. (1992). Can the language of "social maladjustment" in the SED definition be ignored? *School Psychology Review, 21,* 21-22.

Sparrow, S., Cicchetti, D. V., & Balla, D. (1984). *Vineland Social Maturity Scale-Revised.* Circle Pines, MN: American Guidance Service.

Spitzer, R. L., Davies, M., & Barkley, R. A. (1990). The *DSM-III-R* field trial of disruptive behavior disorders. *Journal of the American Academy of Child and Adolescent Psychiatry, 29,* 690-697.

Stanger, C., Achenbach, T. M., & Verhulst, F. C. (in press). Accelerated longitudinal comparison of aggressive versus delinquent behavior. *Development and Psychopathology.*

Stanger, C., MacDonald, V., McConaughy, S. H., & Achenbach, T. M. (1996). Predictors of cross-informant syndromes among children and youths referred for mental health services. *Journal of Abnormal Child Psychology.*

Stattin, H., & Magnusson, D. (1989). The role of early aggressive behavior in the frequency, seriousness, and types of later crime. *Journal of Consulting and Clinical Psychology, 57,* 710-718.

Steingard, R., Biederman, J., Doyle, A., & Sprich-Buckminster, S. (1992). Psychiatric comorbidity in attention deficit disorder: Impact on the interpretation of Child Behavior Checklist results. *Journal of the American Academy of Child and Adolescent Psychiatry, 31,* 449-454.

Stoff, D. M., Pollock, L., Vitiello, B., Behar, D., & Bridger, W. H. (1987). Reduction of 3-H-imipramine binding sites on platelets of conduct disordered children. *Neuropsychopharmacology, 1,* 55-62.

van den Oord, E. J. C. G., Boomsma, D. I., & Verhulst, F. C. (1994). A study of problem behaviors in 10- to 15-year-old biologically related and unrelated international adoptees. *Behavior Genetics, 24,* 193-205.

van den Oord, E. J. C. G., Verhulst, F. C., & Boomsma, D. I. (in press). A genetic study of maternal and paternal ratings of problem behaviors in three-year-old twins. *Journal of Abnormal Psychology.*

Vandiver, T., & Sher, K. J. (1991). Temporal stability of the Diagnostic Interview Schedule. *Psychological Assessment, 3,* 277-281.

Verhulst, F. C., & van der Ende, J. (1992). Six-year stability of parent-reported problem behavior in an epidemiological sample. *Journal of Abnormal Child Psychology, 20,* 595-610.

Walker, L. S., Garber, J., & Greene, J. W. (1991). Somatization symptoms in pediatric abdominal pain patients: Relation to chronicity of abdominal pain and parent somatization. *Journal of Abnormal Child Psychology, 19,* 379-394.

Walker, J. L., Lahey, B. B., Russo, M. F., Christ, M. A. G., McBurnett, K., Loeber, R., Stouthamer-Loeber, M., & Green, S. M. (1991). Anxiety, inhibition, and conduct disorder in children: I. Relations to social impairment. *Journal of the American Academy of Child and Adolescent Psychiatry, 30,* 187-191.

Watson, D. C., & Clark, L. A. (1984). Negative affectivity: The disposition to experience aversive emotional states. *Psychological Bulletin, 96,* 465-490.

Watson, D., Clark, L. A., Weber, K., Assenheimer, J. S., Strauss, M. E., & McCormick, R. A. (1995). Testing a tripartite model: II. Exploring the symptom structure of anxiety and depression in student, adult, and patient samples. *Journal of Abnormal Psychology, 104,* 15-25.

Watson, D., Weber, K., Assenheimer, J. S., Clark, L. A., Strauss, M. E., & McCormick, R. A. (1995). Testing a tripartite model: I. Evaluating the convergent and discriminant validity of anxiety and depression symptom scales. *Journal of Abnormal Psychology, 104,* 3-14.

Wechsler, D. C. (1981). *Wechsler Adult Intelligence Scale–Revised.* New York: Psychological Corporation.

Wechsler, D. C. (1991). *Wechsler Intelligence Scale for Children–Third edition.* San Antonio, TX: Psychological Corporation.

Weinstein, S. R., Noam, G. G., Grimes, K., Stone, K., & Schwab-Stone, M. (1990). Convergence of *DSM-III* diagnoses and self-reported symptoms in child and adolescent inpatients. *Journal of the American Academy of Child and Adolescent Psychiatry, 29,* 627-634.

Weisz, J. R., Donenberg, G. R., Han, S. S., & Kauneckis, D. (1995). Child and adolescent psychotherapy outcomes in experiments and clinics: Why the disparity? *Journal of Abnormal Child Psychology, 23,* 83-106.

Weisz, J. R., Weiss, B., Han, S. S., Granger, D. A., & Morton, T. (1995). Effects of psychotherapy with children and adolescents revisited: A meta-analysis of treatment outcome studies. *Psychological Bulletin, 117,* 450-468.

Wolraich, M. L., Hannah, J. N., Pinnock, T. Y., Baumgaertel, A., & Brown, J. (1996). Comparison of diagnostic criteria for Attention-Deficit Hyperactivity Disorder in a county-wide sample. *Journal of the American Academy of Child and Adolescent Psychiatry, 35,* 319-324.

Woodcock, R. E., & Johnson, M. D. (1989). *Woodcock-Johnson Psychoeducational Battery-Revised.* Hingham, MA: Teaching Resources Corporation.

World Health Organization. (1992). *Mental disorders: Glossary and guide to their classification in accordance with the Tenth Revision of the International Classification of Diseases* (10th ed.). Geneva: Author.

Zahn-Waxler, C., Schmitz, S., Fulker, D., Robinson, J., & Emde, R. (1996). Behavior problems in 5-year-old monozygotic and dizygotic twins: Genetic and environmental influences, patterns of regulation, and internalization of control. *Development and Psychopathology, 8,* 103-122.

Zoccolillo, M. (1993). Gender and the development of conduct disorder. *Development and Psychopathology, 5,* 65-78.

AUTHOR INDEX

SUBJECT INDEX

ABOUT THE AUTHORS

Thomas M. Achenbach is Professor of Psychiatry and Psychology and Director of the Center for Children, Youth, and Families at the University of Vermont. A graduate of Yale, he received his Ph.D. from the University of Minnesota and was a postdoctoral Fellow at the Yale Child Study Center. Before moving to the University of Vermont, he taught at Yale and was a Research Psychologist at the National Institute of Mental Health. He has been a DAAD Fellow at the University of Heidelberg, Germany, an SSRC Senior Faculty Fellow at Jean Piaget's Centre d'Epistemologie Genetique in Geneva, Chair of the American Psychological Association's Task Force on Classification of Children's Behavior, and a member of the American Psychiatric Association's Advisory Committee on the *DSM-III-R*. He is author of *Developmental Psychopathology; Research in Developmental Psychology: Concepts, Strategies, Methods; Assessment and Taxonomy of Child and Adolescent Psychopathology; Empirically Based Taxonomy,* and manuals for the Child Behavior Checklist, Teacher's Report Form, and Youth Self-Report.

Stephanie H. McConaughy is Research Associate Professor in the Department of Psychiatry at the University of Vermont. A graduate of the University of Michigan, she received an M.Ed. in education and Ph.D. in psychology from the University of Vermont. She is a licensed practicing psychologist and a nationally certified school psychologist. She specializes in assessment of children's behavioral and emotional problems and learning disabilities, and serves as a psychological consultant to local school districts. She has presented workshops on child assessment to psychologists and special educators throughout the United States and abroad. Her research has been supported by the National Institute of Education, National Institute on Disability and Rehabilitation Research, National Institute of Mental Health, Spencer Foundation, and W.T. Grant

Foundation. She has published three books and numerous articles and chapters on children's behavioral/emotional and learning problems. She also authored the Vermont Guidelines for Identifying Students Experiencing Emotional-Behavioral Disabilities. She has served as Associate Editor of the *School of Psychology Review* and as Vermont delegate to the National Association of School Psychologists.